ALCHEMY OF DESIRE,
REVOLT & VIOLENCE

ALCHEMY OF DESIRE, REVOLT & VIOLENCE

A Study in Discourses of Sexuality & Violence

VISHNU PATIL

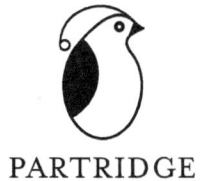

PARTRIDGE

To order additional copies of this book, contact
Partridge India
000 800 10062 62
orders.india@partridgepublishing.com

www.partridgepublishing.com/india

Contents

Dedicated to
My loving mother Umavati
&
Beautiful memories of my father

Acknowledgement

I wish to express my gratitude to my supervisor Dr. Arvind M. Nawale for both his constant support and guidance in formulating this research work and constant encouragement to read and bring about applications of different theories to the texts written by Elkunchwar. I thank him profusely for his patient supervision, considerate critical attention and consistent friendly and helpful disposition throughout the preparation of this research work. He provided me with the critical insight about the genre, which proved a lifelong learning experience. Moreover he has been a tremendous source of inspiration. He is a prolific writer with his huge critical writings and his contribution is promising.

My mother has been a great source of inspiration for me always. Wish my father could see this book. I thank my brother Shankar and *vahini* Lata, sisters Sangita and Anita for their enormous love. I am so happy and delighted to have a wife like Krutika who never tolerated me neglecting my health during my work. She has been a great support without which

I could not have completed my work. She took care of my sweet angel Kavya while I was busy in my work. I thank my friends Dr. Balaji Devkate, Anil Chindhe, Dr. Vijay Matkar, Shashikant Bhosale Dr. Atul Keche and Rajaram Jeve for their love and support.

-Patil Vishnu Wamanrao

Chapter ▌
INTRODUCTION

Mahesh Elkunchwar receives more significance being a notable playwright in the post-independence era in India due to various reasons. There are many opinions and ideas proposed by many thinkers about what exactly went into making of Marathi theatre in particualr and Indian theatre at large.

Sayan Dey in his article declares that artistic talent like that of Elkunchwar was the outcome of certain circumstances that were produced after India received independence. According to Sayan, there was 'artistic confusion' and 'fragmentation' during the period and he continues, "[T]he entire nation was bifurcated over the issue of retaining Indian traditionalism or inheriting western modernism. These theatrical dialectics generated original or synthesized versions of thematic and performative principles" (Dey 18). However there had been more than single stimulus for Elkunchwar to decide on making writing plays his profession on personal and cultural level. The 'singularization' of view about the key factors affecting the development of theatre in India after independence may not be very fruitful as the country does not hold uniformity neither on the level of language nor that of culture and traditions. This fact makes the process more complicated to think on it more systematically and on the other hand it brings about more artistic and innovative form of writing with the uniqueness of experience embedded in the language and the culture of the local.

Elkunchwar banged on the screen with the exhibitions of the experiences which were considered 'taboo' and selected such subject matter that had been an important part of the entire section of the middle class society against the rural backdrop. Agriculture and traditional business were the backbone of economy of the society. It was the period of transition in India at national as well as local level. Economy was being stirred at the levels of development caused by industrial growth, educational advancements and the nature of agricultural prosperity. Elkunchwar becomes representative of the both the typical family stystem in Indian villages with all those family bondages and conflicts and that of the life style affected by more and more urbanization.

There is more than one reason that makes Mahesh Elkunchwar one of the most prominent playwrights in Marathi literary writing after independence. Vijay Tendulkar was at his peak of career and it was watching his play *Mi Jinkalo Mi Harlo!* inspired Elkunchwar to make writing plays as his profession. He wrote the finest plays in Marathi that contributed in bringing about elementary changes in the scenario of Marathi play writing. It is approximately after 1960, the writings of Mardhekar, Gadgil, Tendulkar, Khanolkar and Alekar dealt with new themes and touched upon many new issues and sought clear and bold representation of them in literature. This 'new writing' brought larger dimensions to Marathi literature. They made experiments with forms, themes, narratives techniques and explored new and prohibited areas of human experiences. In this task of exploration, Elkunchwar stands alone with difference to that of traditional and contemporary playwrights. It is so due to the major concern of his plays that deals with such a basic structure of family and society in Maharashtra, touching upon very common human emotions and struggles. What the common lays in his writings is distinctive nature of philosophy he propagates. It is why Dr. Kamlesh says that "ethos, core and concern of Elkunchwar are different" and he is primarily a philosopher.

Elkunchwar has strong belief regarding what mainly constitutes the process of perception of a play i.e. writing, reading, watching a play being performed and a play being performed by actors and their perception of the play. He elaborates his stand regarding it in the annexure to the play *Wada Chirebandi* entitled *Maza Ajwarcha Natyapravas*. Though there has been for a long period of time a debate about what constitutes as a prominent core of an art among text, context, author and reader, he thinks it is not the author, nor the audience but the actor who is more prominent; its his/her body that labours to express human mind. To search for the mind is the real performance. Human mind is limitless and there is no end to the agony of the mind. Performances must be executed to find out the depth of the agony of human mind.

This view of Elkunchwar bears more significance and controversy as it passes judgment challenging the authorial 'supremacy', contextual relevance, and importance of audience's perception of the play. Elkunchwar is one of the few dramatists and critics who hold this view. It bears the authenticity on many grounds as actors are the most important medium that brings about the realization of author's ideas to the audience. Randolph Goodman adds to the role of other factors on the stage saying, "To bring a script successfully to life on the stage requires the skill and artistry of many professional practitioners – director; actors; scene, costume, and lighting designers; and occasionally a composer and choreographer – all working in concert" (Goodman vii).

This is perhaps more intelligible to a dramatist to recognize how his/her play is being transformed into performance and how meaning is more orineted to the actors and their ways of expressions. It becomes more clear to the author when he/she comes to know how there has been vital change in the meaning creation between what the author implied and what the actor expressed. It could be happening in case of play writing only. As other forms of writing may not give this idea to an author, a dramatist receives more time to contemplate and realize the transformation as he/she could sit in a theatre and watch her/his play being performed. Elkunchwar seems to be more impressed by this phenomenon. It has a vital perception to think over as there have been multiple issues taken into consideration about as what constitutes the making of a play or a text. Though Elkunchwar talks about the significance of actors who bring about a world of change in meaning with the manners in which they enact a play, he considers positively all elements that offer their contribution in the making of a text, which could be listed as author and her/his milieu, the time, gender, politics, culture and history. At the minutest level if one attempts to observe, it is highly possible to find how the smallest gesture on the part of an actor changes the meaning of the course of the action. It builds entirely new formation of cultural associations and changes the whole schemata of the play planned by the author. Malyaban Chattopadhyay's article entitled "A Historical Study of Ancient Indian Theatre – Communication in the Light of *Natyashastra*" writes about ideological perspectives as far as presentations by actors on the stage are concerned. It becomes clear that possible effects of the free expressions by the actors on the stage, were recognized and it was clearly stated 'to control' performances in country and Malyaban thinks that such strategy of controlling was formulated as the performers were 'good communicators' and they could be threats to powers of the state. Malyaban registers an important idea from the *Natyasastra* translated by Adya Rangacharya. It says, "Things which are not stated here should be learnt by attentively watching the talking and behavior of the people and should be used in performance" (quoted in Chattopadhyay 12).

Many a times, this view of Elkunchwar has instigated many discussions among the literary circles in Maharashtra, and occupied larger space in media too. However, it is essential to locate Elkunchwar in a tradition of which he is one of the 'alterers' as far as Indian drama in general and Marathi theatrical writings in particular are concerned. This tradition at both the levels does not seem to be receiving single stimulus for it to lead in a particular direction. Colonialism and postcolonial conditions could be an umbrella term to gather whole course of process. It was not an easy job for the Indians people to cope up with the change after independence. It had been complex phenomenon for them as they live under control and subjugation of the British people for more than a century. Before the arrival of British people, there had been different aristocratic regions where they fought for soverignity of their status and their people. It was the memory Indians had; the struggle for independence was a vital phenomenon that united India in better way. It was for the first time, whole country lead by Mahatma Gandhi, was united as a nation and declared to be a free nation and democracy was established. This course of history has more impact on the life of common people. In addition to this, the technological, industrial and economical advancement triggered multifarious effects on the traditions, cultures, rituals and family system in India. Economy forms the base of every change in social life.

As a result, a researcher has to consider these issues more systematically in order to understand basic nature of texts produced in India. Prof. T.M.J. Indamohan in his paper entitled "Post-Colonial Writing – Trends in English Drama" considers *Reflection* of nationalism in post colonial drama in liberated nations as a form of "resuscitating the respective nations' socio-cultural and political dignity from the imperial compression" (Indramohan 5). For him it is a matter of psychological and identity crisis. He concludes his paper by saying that the post colonial plays "do not theorise any particular aspect but articulate the categories of social and psychic identity and their labile new deployments across the ideological spectrum and it is discipline stands away from the superpower's hold and carve a niche of their own in the history of race, culture and politics" (Indramohan 5).

Cravings for identity were a visible and natural trait that could be easily seen among the countries receiving political freedom. However all attempts to recover from the 'colonized mind' and asserting identity of their own were never devoid of exhibitions of the richness of the traditions they had. For a country like India, it was supported by and correlated with religious rituals, traditional festivals and folk arts. With the passage of time, the intensity of nationalism, explicit exhibition and assertion of identity through various forms of literature and arts started to ebb away gradually. It took for a while for Indians to make out the design of their country which had been changed due to certain course of events like religious riots, political and democratic upheavals, and constitutional provisions for under privileged people of India, establishment of *Panchayat Raj* and implementation of Five Year Plans. The division of the country among states on the basis of language and considerable growth of population has distinctive impact on the feelings of nationalism of the country and psychology of linguistic compartments still continues to exist.

G. P. Deshpande's following view makes the complexity of the division of period visible. He writes in his introduction to his book entitled *Modern Indian Drama: An Anthology*, "Indian theatre however seemed to pursue a different path. It was *not* post-colonial. It was not post-modern either. It seemed to hark back to tradition and the ethnic. It seemed to celebrate the 'Indian' more than any other form of writing in India" (Deshpande xiv, xv).

Gradually with development of industrialization that was more associated with the intensive growth in population and consumerism, India started getting divided into two major sections i.e. rural and urban. There were more reasons to the movement of masses from rural area to the cities than that of employment. Both the places have developed a distinctive nature of lifestyle. The residents of the places have certain magnitude of psychological orientations that are characteristically different from each other. In an extreme manner, Arvind Adiga mentions village as 'area of darkness' and city as 'area of light' in his Booker award winning novel *The White Tiger*. The protagonist Balram tell Jiabao that "a man can be good in city if he wants to be but in village he doesn't have this choice" (Adiga 98) and he adds to it saying that this difference between the two Indias is 'the choice'. *The White Tiger* could be taken here as one of the finest examples that represent Indian life so well depicted as divided among the two sections. Besides it, it is a picture of developing India presented by a person who experienced age long poverty and had been victimized by the different systems in India. This view however brings us one idea as stated earlier that a certain phenomenon like that of a typical writing cannot be studied in isolation. It has to be judged in multiple ways as there are many visible and invisible factors that go in making of a text, its perception, its realization and its popularity as well.

In this way, we can very roughly point out how the chronological order may run beginning with nationalism, politically inspired identity crisis, glorification of traditions and confrontation with modern ways of living, increasing complexities of relationships, fragmentation of traditional social structures, and institutions like marriage and family and identity crisis within a society and institutions. The chronology leads to what generally is called as modern Indian drama. Daxa Thakor thinks that it as a "combination of tradition and modernity where tradition is equated with old outdated ideas and beliefs and customs and practices and modernity with progress and new ideas" (Thokar 2).

It is interesting to observe how dramatic critical writings in India have two distinctive levels. One deals with the production of dramatic writing in vernaculars and its translation that enabled the writing across the borders of the states and reach out not only to the other states in India but also abroad. At another level, dramatic production originally in English like that of Mahesh Dattani is evaluated. Each language in India has its own tradition of dramatic writing in form of folk art or the other, like other form of literary genre. Translation was and is a spectacular phenomenon that functions on two levels in an affirmative way; it carries the literature of one vernacular language to English speaking people and it also facilitates authors writing in their own languages and thus maintaining their originality, best representation of their culture, social issues and conflicts in their mothertongue. As a post colonial 'decolonization of mind' project, it disqualifies the unnecessary burden of learning or knowing English for expression of one's ideas.

It also becomes essential to observe vastness of literary production in India so divided in roughly three levels i.e. vernacular, translated and originally written in English. However, one might find how it is only few writings and writers who are often quoted while writing a survey of Indian drama. It tends to prompt any common reader to make out the smaller arena of Indian dramatic writing. However, this view should not ignore the rich tradition of dramatic writing and performance in India that had been as old as the culture itself. It is rich with expressions, concerns and ways of presentation. A book entitled *Indian Drama in English* edited by Kaustav Chakraborty contains articles on dramatic works of Tagore, Vijay Tendulkar, Girish Karnad, Mahasweta Devi, Mahesh Dattani, Habib Tanvir, Indira Parthsarathy, Asif Currimbhoy and Badal Circar. It gives an idea that less than six states in India have produced significant dramatic writing. He concludes his "Introduction: Representative Playwrights of Indian English Drama" with the following vague note on the scope English drama in India:

> Writing is only one aspect of the play; the other predominant one is the performance. Does English theatre, then, exclude the majority of the populance, an audience that would otherwise have easily received a play in their own mother tongue? This is the crux of the problem that poses the major obstacle for Indian dramatic performances in English. However, with decades of English education in India, both in schools and in universities, the country is home to the largest English-knowing population in the world. Hence, there is still a large potential audience for plays written in or translated into English (Chakraborty 18).

In his article entitled "A Short Survey of Contemporary Indian Drama", Dr. M. H. Khandagale in the book *Reflection of the Changing Indian Society in Indian English Drama*, initially makes few reference to historical background of Indian tradition of drama writing and different folk form of dramatic presentations in different states and then mentions Tagore, Aurobindo and Harindranath Chattopadhyaya as significant playwrights during pre-independence era. However, his list of contemporary drama only consists of Currimbhoy, Dharmavir Bharati, Badal Circar, Mohan Rakesh, Tendulkar and Karnad and it completes his survey. However he points out few thematic concerns that hold together the literary production by the authors. He says, "One of the things which profoundly unite them is their mutually complementary treatment of the problematic of contemporary Indian subjectivity on the various axes of gender, sexuality, history, tradition, class and socio-cultural change" (Khandagale 14-15).

The major reason for a limited and restricted list of contemporary dramatists in English and in translation is due to less serious drama writing and lack of development of culture of theatrical and professional performances of plays. As far as Marathi theatrical writing or performances are concerned, Pune and Mumbai were once few of the most outstanding producers of professional plays and the cities also had a good number of theatre goers. It was during 1900 to 1920 and 1970s & 1980s and since then there had been many declining trends.

Elkunchwar forms his very crucial role as a dramatist in Marathi writing and joins the modern Marathi dramatists like Vijay Tendulkar, Satish Alekar and C.T. Khanolkar. With the translation of his plays, he became one of the most widely read dramatists in India. Dr. Supriya Pendhari is right to observe that the emergence of Tendulkar, Elkunchwar, Satish Alekar and Khanolkar was of a literary 'revolt' sort against the traditional playwriting on the both levels thematic and structural. It was mainly dominated by the authors like V.V. Shirvadkar, Vasant Kanetkar, Madhusudan Karlekar, P. B. Bhave, Bal Kolhatkar, S. G. Sathe, Vidyadhar Gokhale and Purushottam Darvhekar. If we see the thematic concerns of the plays like *Silence! The Court is in Session*, *Sakharam*

Binder, Vultures, Ghashiram Kotwal, Chanakya, Vishnugupt, Mahanirvan, Begum Barve, Suryast, Vasanakand, Atmakatha, Garbo, etc.; we can realize how they were distinctively different from the old traditional plays. They essentially contain a voice of revolt that is asserted with a purpose that mainly intends to depict realism of gender discrimination, religious conflict and psychological problems. They rather incorporated the element of literary revolt and controversy in their plays like *Ghashiram Kotwal, Sakharam Binder* by Tendulkar and *Garbo* and *Wasanakand* by Elkunchwar.

The present study concentrates on certain elements like 'desire', 'revolt' and 'violence' in the select plays of Mahesh Elkunchwar. It however does become a part of a larger picture that contributes in making certain writing in Marathi as modern one. Though the themes or traits like sexuality and violence are few of the major issues dealt with on the stage, they have been embedded with other issues to mainly economic, social and ideological structures. There are myriad forces that function in ways which can never satisfactorily be adjusted to our predetermined categories like binary oppositions. It is also essential to recognize that such forces are not entirely independent. They are limited in a particular structure which could exist in a certain way at a certain period of time. For example dramatists like Shirvadkar, Khanolkar, Tendulkar and Elkunchwar have a type of literary production in a form of dramatic writing that does not limit itself to limited arena of social structure they are part of or nor is there always a constant effort for making their writings politically correct and intentionally fortified or manufactured.

Authors like Tendulkar and Elkunchwar do attempt to present artistically realism which is both visible and invisible in the structures of various relationships. In a general sense, this act by any author becomes a particular form of a 'gesture' that does not necessarily go with the common perception of reality. Such gestures are always probing and encroaching the established 'ways of seeing'. It could be called as a revolt in a certain sense. With this understanding, it becomes necessary to realize that the use of word revolt is manifold and as far as this research work is concerned, it is used in both the ways i.e. revolt in general sense and revolt in literary sense which could be written as 'literary revolt'. What difference does matter between the two is that of origin and inspiration of the revolt.

According to Supriya Pendhari, typical interest of an established author is nurtured on the interest of common people. "There comes a time in course of event of writing that such authors produce literature of a typical kind which would be appreciated by common readers and audiences" (Pendhari 1). There exist a tradition of perception of literature on two levels i.e. readers or audiences and authors. The former lacks creativity as a response to the improper selection of subject matter, repetition of same subjects and sacrifice of virtue and creativity for the sake of appreciation of common readers or audiences. The later takes it more seriously and attempts for systematic responses in the form of creative writing. As there exists no natural or supernatural system that maintains moderations of proper proportional distribution of justice to a subject and appreciation for innovations and new ways of 'seeing' or 'writing', the literary revolt becomes necessary as it is the only way out for the people with innovations and creativity. However the established tradition and literary circle do not allow the change to take place. It prepares such a literary system which is maintained by various bodies and institutions that look after its perpetual existence and cultural, social and political circumstances become favourable to it and protect it.

Literary revolt does give birth to a literature which has more sensibility, creativity, new world of experience, new aestheticism and variety of outlook. This process however is not easy one. It takes time to establish itself and there remains always a threat of suppression and becoming outcast. The test of appreciation by common readers becomes more essential at initial stages too. The revolt could be hopeless if it is not supported with proper and systematic literary production of higher kind. The vividness of certain superficial aspects in more vague and more trivial way reduces the life of the revolt. *Dalit* literature is called as a literature of revolt and protest. It marks a very productive and rich period in Marathi as well as in Indian literature. Though it had its roots in the age long sufferings and suppression which is of more than mere literary experience, there are common and universal elements that form a base for all literature of revolt. It is why Hemangi Bhagwat identifies the *dalit* theatre as representative of all the suppressed in her article "Dalit Theatre: A Theatre of Protest". She concludes saying that *dalit* theatre "can be called as the theatre of the 'proletariat' in the truest sense of the term. Hence its significance as 'a social theatre' is to be acknowledged' (Bhagwat 384).

The literature of revolt is labeled as a threat to the culture. It is feared that such type of revolt may cause damage to whole literary traditions and will limit its area of expression. Literature of revolt always leaves its water mark not only in a certain period of literary production but also it adds a chapter to the whole history of mankind. It basically strengthens the culture and also it brings revival to it. Each new trait in a culture is a sort of revolt in its miniature. Perhaps it is a protest and revolt that bring about richness and strength to any kind of literary tradition and culture. Revolt becomes a very important concept in this regard. It is actually identical to the process of development of human civilization. When Datta Bhagat in his article entitled "Marathi Natak: 1975 to 2000" questions the rigidity of unchanging nature of Marathi drama, it suggests the validity of literary revolt. He says, "Before independence Marathi play writing acted politics and socialism and continued the same after independence. Security of them would be threatened was the main fear for them; after independence there had been fearless atmosphere. Then why had there been no picture of real politics in Marathi plays?" (Bhagat 111)

Literary revolt has its limited field of experience. It takes place within the boundaries of experience among the community of creative writing. It becomes an act by a certain group of authors that create typical form of writing that does not follow the norms and style introduced and established by traditional mainstream authors. The inspirations for such act by new authors are of purely creative and artistic nature. It has inspirations of broader sense that act beyond the common desires for popularity and making money. It becomes a tool for bringing about a change in common taste for literature and introducing whole new world of experiences and realities. However, it is articulated based on the world of reality created by the existing authors through their writings and it acts mainly for what T. S. Eliot calls 'correction of taste' in his essay Tradition and Individual Talent. Thus literary revolt becomes an aggressive gesture in terms of form and style. It firmly believes in efficacy and effectiveness of new ways of presentations, representations and expressions. It works against the known fact that certain successful formulae do function in bringing about certain positive responses from readers and audiences. This act of literary revolt at a juncture is an act of risk taking in economic and professional sense.

On the other hand, revolt in general sense means the response to a particular culture or development in a culture in a way that could be aggressive, intimidating, hostile and non-cooperative as well; it receives its origins in multiple sources like society, institutions, religion, human relationships, economic structures, political categories and systems, history, geographical orientations and disparities, technologically driven changes, environmental changes, etc.

In the modernist writings of playwrights like Dattani who writes purely in English, Mahasweta Devi, Badal Circar, Datta Bhagat, Sanjay Pawar, Tendulkar, Elkunchwar, etc. have more issues and concerns of unconventional and illegitimate nature at thematic levels in their representations on stage. Sexual issues like prostitution, incest, child abuse, extramarital affairs, rape, violent issues like communal violence, riots, domestic violence, feticide, disaster, political violence, Naxalism, murder, suicide and social and historical issues like castism, slavery, gender discrimination, exploitation, psychological disorders, etc. are the thematic body of plays of modern Indian playwrights through which three aspects are highlighted. One being the representation of realism and the second the outcry for transformation and change in the existing system and the third is activism.

Selection of issues of sexuality and violence on the stage has the element of literary revolt as well. However, it has roots more importantly in social, political and cultural orientation rather than purely literary inspirations. The inspirations of Tendulkar and Elkunchwar for writing plays differ radically. Elkunchwar's literary forte right from inspiration writing plays to the selection of theme, subject, form and style is purely a literary inspiration. Though Elkunchwar admits that his has been literary inspiration to writing as his profession, it is essential to recognize that such singularity does not always consist of uniformity of entity called literature. There are various factors that go into making of world of one's literature.

Elkunchwar's plays have imagism as their strongest point. It is with the effective use of various images and symbols; he succeeds in presenting a structure of story imbedded with multiple possible meaning having very effective touch of metaphysics and philosophy. He seems to be representing the eternal conflict of human being caught between the trajectories like desire and satisfaction. The conflict has multiple culminations. Elkunchwar very skillfully catches them in their typical forms in various contexts. Existential crises are one of major traits of his complete writing. They are visible in the plays like *Reflection* and *Desire in the Rocks*. It is with all the complexity of existence of human being, the inclination of events towards absurdity becomes obvious. Murder of Garbo could be the best example of such act. Treatment to the subjects like desire, revolt, violence, existentialism and absurdity by Elkunchwar is never devoid of a philosophy that is mainly affected by the culture of the local, personal history and inability of resolving psychological dilemmas and confusions.

Elkunchwar's imagism and symbolism succeed in conveying the idea of futility of human desire. It also succeeds in presenting subtle satire on various trends, traditions and practices in society. Sometimes it seems that it is a reflection of the authors mind; his struggle to make out the meaning of various events and conflicts in life. The gravity of Elkunchwar's ways of presentation of such human emotional crises seems to be suggesting the redundancy of human emotional, psychological and philosophical queries against the farfetched technological and industrial advancements. The social milieu depicted in his plays has a very positive impact on readers and audiences particularly from the rural and urban area of Maharashtra. It is perhaps the most authentic and effective representation of rural parts in Maharashtra where there exist a typical system of interrelations among people of various caste and religion. Elkunchwar does not only succedd in bringing about the representation of conflict and intensity of the experience of the locale but also builds a set of the culture that each reader and audience feels a close association with it. It appeals to the both categories of the readers and audience i.e. rural and urban. For the urban, it has become a memory that is not so distant and Elkunchwar with his plays like *Old Stone Mansion*, *Pond* and

Apocalypse brings a vivid picture of the life from dismantling social and family system in rural parts of Maharashtra.

The social and family system that mainly depends on agriculture, has been crucially affected by low rainfall, scarcity of water and droughts. Each year brings a test to the patience and hopefulness of farmers and to those whose livelihood depends on agriculture. Elkunchwar's depiction of degrading conditions at rural area especially in *Wada Trilogy* is an attempt to present a picture of helpless conditions of people caught among uninformed division of economic development and watertight compartments that does not leave space of mobility of rural area. The complexity and wilderness of decision making after losing the basement of age long traditions that formed the very basis of their psyche, and inability to gauge and adopt the technological driven changes and value system are depicted at various levels by the dramatist.

The *modus operandi* of almost all of Elkunchwar's plays could be related to the three types of reality as proposed by Lacan i.e. the imaginary, the symbolic and the real. Imaginary refers to the reality that everyone conceives and it plays an important role in deciding the world view of a person. Imaginary is images which are so strong that they are real. Though they still remain image, they are so strong as to have vital impact on human mind and thus they are real. The symbolic reality refers to the kind of reality which is already fixed like that of patriarchy and the real refers to the fact how reality itself is formed. It is reality of reality. It does not refer to a transcendental meaning, meaning final kind of reality. It just refers to the construction of reality in a certain situation and time that is a construction of certain forces and 'ways of seeing'. Most of his plays' main course is based on the three issues. The understanding of the course of events is essential in order to understand the meaning of actions of the characters in Elkunchwar's plays. The idea of reality is very crucial in human life. It is a complicated phenomenon which forms the base of human experience without most of the times, for an individual, realizing the workings of it. It has multi layers to distinguish among what one thinks about oneself; what one thinks what others think about him/her; and what others really think about him/her. Every human gesture or action is affected by one of the above mentioned ones. On the other levels, it has to work with the two categories mentioned before i.g. the symbolic and the real. The three realities have world of web of complex interrelations in a person's thinking capacity. They function in accordance with the systematic maintenance of equilibrium of all elements that support a glorification of the self and also a perception that the person is normal and wise. The standards of such normality and wisdom are predetermined. As long as glorification, standards of normality and wisdom are felt distinctively, there emerges no problem for an individual. As one cannot manage the course of events which possess external force beyond one's control, it is quite difficult to realize and manage the complex structure of effects caused by imbalance among the views on the three categories of reality. They are never devoid of the issues that actually form the base of psyche of the community or the person. Religion, gender, caste, ideology, desire, institutions, social systems, etc are few of the frequent issues that form relevance and reference for the certain culmination of a conflict. For instance, murder of Garbo by Shrimant in *Garbo*, suicide by Lalita in *Desire in the Rocks*, suicide by Chandrashekhar in *Sultan*, extramarital affairs of Aai in *As One Descardeth the Old Clothes...*, murder of Amrit in *Party* and suicide by Anand in *Holi*, etc. basically have the reasons among the conflicts caused by the disturbances to the different forms of reality.

Lacan calls the symbolic, the ideal or imaginary and the real as the three registers of human reality. He stressed many times since 1950s, the idea of the symbolic. It is understood as the network, social, cultural, linguistic milliue, into which a child is born. It is why Lacan always says that language is there before the actual moment of birth of the child and it will act on the whole of its existence. Lacan assigns more importance to the symbolic as he thinks it plays a vital role in human experience of significations. While speaking about the ideal or imaginary, he says that "there is an identification which is both beyond and in a sense prior to the identification with the image: a symbolic identification with a signifying element. He calls it is an identification with the ideal" (Leader 44). He reformulated the concept of the real several times in his works. For him the real is simply that isn't symbolized. It is that which is excluded from the symbolic. It resists the symbolic absolutely. In this way, for us reality exists only between two levels i.g. symbolic and imaginary. The real is precisely that for Lacan, which is excluded from reality. It is a kind of boundary of what is without meaning and which we fail to situate or explore.

This excessive stress on the idea of reality is essential as far as the present research work is concerned. It is precisely the idea of reality with its three registers that matters in forming a world view and determines the course of action for each individual. It could be a major tool to understand the nature of acts, events, conflicts in the issues like desire, revolt and violence in the plays of Mahesh Elkunchwar.

Sultan was the first one act play of Elkunchwar. It has four symbolic characters named Rajshekhar, Doctor, Swami and Julie along with the tiger named Sultan in the cage. The play is an attempt on the part of the playwright to depict 'vanity of human wishes' for ultimate satisfaction. Elkunchwar builds up the characters like Rajshekhar who faces the void of human existence, Doctor whose world of emotions and significance is limited to his self only, Swami is a hypocrite who assumes satisfaction in superficial realization and Julie is always busy in embellishment of her body. Death becomes a central event of the play. Rajshekhar commits suicide. Before he shoots himself, he shoots the tiger Sultan as well. The complex structure of registers of reality gets complicated in determining the fulfillment of desires and it has many culminations among which revolt and violence are the most prominent ones. Elkunchwar present symbolic and imaginary in a certain form. The four characters along with the tiger are symbolic. Julie's love for beautification of her body being a woman, Swami's expected indulgence in superficial realization of self control and satisfaction and Doctor's world that is limited to himself suggest the symbolic being perceived and resulting in the ideal. It becomes an essential condition for them or any human being for that matter, to survive in the situation. The two registers contain a sense of sustainability in them which assures continuity of existence and avoid conflicts. Rajshekhar's restlessness and realization of absurdity and meaninglessness of human existence leads him to uniformity of his mind that strongly formed a sense of meaning between the symbolic and the ideal. The loss of it leads him to commit suicide. It is precisely the conflict arising from the symbolic and imaginary for Rajshekhar that leads him to violent end. His ego does not offer him rationalization of his actions when he was restless and distrust or loss of faith in things with certain meaning brings about break to positivity of thought that advocates life. The real is beyond the symbolic and the ideal. It could be related to the ideas of Dr. Sandhya Amrute when she says, "The thoughts of death of Rajshekhar result into the death of him. It has its origin in the thought when he believes that there is no escape from this system without death and if at all there is happiness and satisfaction, it could be state after death"(Amrute 173).

In a particular sense, the symbolic traps psyche of an individual in a certain manner that does not allow making any change as it is predetermined and there is hardly anything an individual can do about it. It percolates into becoming the ideal. The ideal always has an alteration on the individual level.

Naresh from *Zumbar* meaning chandelier has deeper levels of dissatisfaction and he probes deeper into the philosophical question of certain meaning of life and events in it. The idea of beauty is artificial and culture specific. The chandelier symbolizes the world view of beauty and it is an attraction for everybody. For Naresh, the reality of life on the symbolic and imaginary levels ceases to exist on accounts of realization of meaninglessness of life on various levels. Though the play does not end in violence, it has turn of events which is not considered as normal. Of course, normality itself is symbolic. The psychological conflict that Naresh faces is in direct connection with the symbolic and ideal order of the world. He struggles for his whole life to achieve the success he has reached to. It was the result of his firm faith in the order. It sustained his beliefs till the time when he realized the ultimate outcome of all the fame and achievements in his life. For him, it signifies nothing. He asks several questions to himself about meaning and purpose of life. He thinks if there is no such exact reason for anything, the whole existence becomes meaningless. This idea makes him restless and faces fragmentation of belief in the order.

It is interesting to watch how in most of Elkunchwar's plays, confict results into a sort of negativity and denial to existing system. Violence and death become his favourite choices. In both the cases of Rajshekhar and Naresh, the dramatist has tried to suggest the possibilities of realization of reality that has philosophical background. Both the protagonists have renunciation of worldly pleasure and it in case of Rajshekhar is renunciation of his life as well. There is a closure formed by Rajshekhar that denies all possibilities for life as he gets entangled in the web of thoughts of meaninglessness of life.

No solace of certainty is provided to him. He becomes any individual on the earth, who comes to the realization of futility of human life. There are several reasons to the denial to the 'normal' course of life and life itself after realization of the futility. It becomes only possible escape for an individual especially in case of self destruction as other options are closed down. Agonizing mind develops many psychological pains that are literally realized and felt by an individual. It conceives death as an ultimate escape from the trouble. The thought is assisted by ideas of áfter life thoughts' that are mainly influenced by religion. In case like that of Naresh, it becomes a sudden loss of interest for any kind of attachment. The mind does not feel the bondages of relationships and their web of interdependence. The very base of all endeavors, which is desire, is lost.

In *Eka Mhataryach Khun*, Elkunchwar continues the strange inclination towards the idea of death. The symbolism is vivid. The four characters represent certain tendencies and class in the society. However, course of event makes the plot more complex and invites multiple layers of meanings. It is in this one act play Elkunchwar depicts a symbolism of social imbalances. It is unlike the dilemma of Rajshekhar and Naresh, a conflict felt at social level where a class, gender and a creed are slaved and whole canvas of life becomes a desert. There is an old man who has tied two men and a woman with a single rope and dragging them to a prison. Concept of revolt is at the centre in this play. Elkunchwar effectively shows how it becomes very difficult for an individual to fight back the visible agents controlling one's freedom. Revolt could be of two types. One way could be being indifferent and remaining passive thus registering non-operation to the system and secondly responding back violently and face the culminations. In any form of change at social or political level, there has to be certain stages. Foremost is the realization of slavery and subjugation; secondly it is expression of feelings against the situation devoid of any activism. Activism becomes necessary and it perhaps always includes violent responses. The two men and a woman initially express their objections through songs and singing. Then they try to control the old man physically and abuse him orally but fail. Eventually they kill him. Elkunchwar through this course of events signifies the subjugation in society in multiple levels. The voices that resist the oppression are heard in low level in certain context of cultural productions. Attempts are made to subvert the system or abuse it as to distort its forces. Sometimes complete annihilation is sought. When the trio kills the old man, they visualize that it had been evil course of event and as a result they will be perished too. It seems to be a realization on the part of the three characters of their futile existence on the deserted land. They still does not receive any meaningful alternative way of living. Elkunchwar seems to be stressing the idea of necessity of certain forceful domination of a system and eradication of such ways could also be a self destruction. However, what is mainly signified through this is that certain logical and reasonable actions of human beings do not necessarily always receive positive results. For it, there should have been alternative arrangements and human mind should be able to articulate the possibility of certain culminations. Thus Elkunchwar addresses the need of philosophically strong base for every kind of change one wishes to bring about.

His one act play entitled *Ek Osad Gaon* written in 1969 is commentary on

> [H]uman life, making realize a constant shadow of death, looking for the gist of human releationships amidst its complexity, enability of guessing, mysticism, longings and showing deep craving of human wishes... Written in a symbolic manner, Elkunchwar expains the views about life and death through the poetic conversation between two characters" (Pendhari 148-49).

The play falls in line with the plays discussed above. A woman is sitting on heap of soil weaving with wool. It is a village with lot of deserted mansions. There comes an ascetic in the village and there takes place a poetic conversation between the two and through this conversation, Elkunchwar present a new disntinctive form of one act play. P. N. Paranjape comments on this aspect of the play and says,

> "...through the images of the woman, the ascetic, one deserted village, the play as a long poem goes on becoming deeper with meaning in search of self. 'Woman', 'weaving', 'leaves' and 'flowers' in the design, etc. become meaningful images. The way Elkunchwar has tried to make the dialogue poetic is convincing' (quoted in Pendhari 149).

Both the characters have deep levels of life experiences. The woman has accepted the course of life with all its redundance. On the other hand, the ascetic is deeply moved by the thoughts of renunciation. His solitary life has strong devotion towards his principles of ascetics. He is caught and beaten badly after he is wrongly convicted of theft. He is released when it realized that he did not steal anything. Eventually, he decides to have no attachment with anyone or anything. The woman who has accepted boredom of life in the form of weaving falls in love with the ascetic and offers him the shawl she has woven. But he refuses to accept it. This multiplicity of image acts in finer way to suggest how she surrenders herself to him with all she has in her life. The hermit, who does not accept this invitation, refuses to fall for the superficial attraction of worldly life. It becomes a revolt on the part of the ascetic against the common attitude in the society, the cultural traits and deeper cravings of ego for desire fulfillment.

These experiences are very close to the rural life of India and rural life experience in the country is perhaps the most valuable one as it forms the larger part of the country. The issues Elkunchwar deals with are of general as well as specific nature. Though the setting of the plays like *Ek Osad Gaon, Eka Mhataryacha Khun, Wada Triology, Desire in the Rocks*, etc is with rural background, the experience and conflicts faced by the characters are of universal nature. So it becomes difficult to believe in what Deshpande G. P says in his preface to *Modern Indian Drama: An Anthology* published by the Sahitya Akademi,

> It is possible to argue … this "ethnic" element in theatre does give us some brilliant, dazzling moments of theatre-experience; the questions remain if this could at all be the modern India's theatre. A modern, urban Indian who constitutes our principle (proscenium) theatre audience may not be in interested in it in a sustained way because these plays do not relate to his experience; let alone making sense of it (Deshpande xvi).

Elkunchwar himself admits that there are images in the plays like *Zumbar* and *Sultan* which have brought in with certain magnitude which is not natural and it has been an exercise with systematic attempts. However he tells it is not the case with *Holi*. The image of *Holi* fire is very strong in the play. It suggests the revolt of two sorts. It is ourtburst of young generation towards the authoratative domination of the older generation and secondly it is reinforcement of new ideas and violent response as to topple it upside down. Vijaya Mehata a renowned critic and director has special consideration for the play *Holi* by Elkunchwar and she thinks as she writes in the foreword of the second volume of *Collected Plays of Mahesh Elkunchwar* that in 1970 Elkunchwar got in the mainstream of theatre with his two one-act plays *Sultan* and *Holi*. He was very young then. She continues writing that "[F]rom Mahesh's earlier writings, *Holi* went on to become – and still remains-the most path-breaking experiment on many counts. It captured the restlessness and tragic frustration of students on a campus, an experience deeply felt by Mahesh as a young lecturer in Nagpur University" (Mehta xi).

In *Holi* there are students from different strata of society living in the college hostel. They have variety of experience pertaining to religion, caste, ideology, family background, and philosophy. They have a developed sense of right to choose, right to speak and oppose. They have clear ideas and independent thoughts for life. There is also a group of students like Shrivastav, Anand, Ranjeet, Lalu, Taimur, Gopal, Madhav, Thakur, Banerji, Vasanta, Patel, Pandey, Mumy, Kunda, etc. The protest by students against the college's act of not declaring a holiday on *Holi* festival and making them attend a program organized by the college and suicide by Anand, are the major incidents in the play. Both the incidents have different layers of meanings. It is a shock for all the students that their bullying Anand for informing their names to the principal results in death of Anand. Through this one act play, Elkunchwar has succeeded in showing the deep layers in human psyche that are vividly active and can instigate many responses including that of violent ones. What matters in the one act play on level of impression and effect is the solid and firm combination of events and a course of events that produces a finer impact on readers and audience.

It is outstanding depiction of revolt, desire (Anand's homosexual attraction towards Shrivastav) and violence in the form of suicide by Anand. Right from its subject matter to the spontaneous revolt from the young students, bring ideas to the readers and audience that Elkunchwar is attempting to present the need and possibility for a change that must take place. However it is not the only change that is to be brought about on only political and social levels but it however is wished to be at deeper levels of psyche and philosophy. Purnima Kulkarni looks at the play from different perspectives. In her article entitled "Subalterns Speak in Mahesh Elkunchwar's *Holi*", she writes that "[t]he play ends in a catastrophic state due to institutionalized heterosexism" and according to her "the discrimination against them (homosexuals) is often translated into violence" (Kulkarni 219).

While bringing critical perspectives from Lacan, Sayan Dey writes about *Holi* in the following way explaining the two stages as proposed by Lacan and its relevance to the acts of the students. He writes,

> The semiotic stage is the first state of human were … not enough matured to communicate in an appropriate, definite form. The increase in age develops in the child the ability to understand and communicate his own thoughts and ideas which he experiences around. This transformation is interpreted as an imposition on behalf of the society as it forces an individual to lose the state for ignorance and innocence and is almost pushed into the symbolic stage. Individuals violating this norm will be either forced into or exterminated from the existing social order and this is what happens with Lalu in the play (Dey 21-22).

Elkunchwar perhaps is one of the greatest dramatists in India, who takes his writing as his passion and firmly believes that it is not only the subject matter that makes a piece of writing truly good and effective but also it is the compactness of what is presented on the stage. Less number of characters that play crucial role in his plays is the part of his art that provides meaningful gist of incidents and content of the course of incidents by using various techniques. It is perhaps the most beautiful aspect of his writing that he provides necessary information about the history and contemporary consciousness through dialogues and flashback techniques. The beauty of it mainly lies in the style in which it is presented naturally.

Yatanaghar is one of his one act plays. There are only two major characters i.e. Baby and Kamal. Baby is physically challenged and she cannot walk. The reason behind her deformity is her father who tried to abort her unsuccessfully and she is born handicapped. Memory and flashback techniques are effective in the play to provide readers and audience necessary information about background. *Yatanaghar* meaning a torture house becomes an image of a human life which is tormented by memory, helplessness and lack of happiness. Home which means a solace for every person, for Baby, it has turned into a nightmare due to the devastating memories she has to live with. She hates her parents when she realizes that they tried to kill her. She develops attractions towards her brother Ramesh. It has layers of desires for him. Kamal takes care of her but she does not like her love for her brother as she has developed feelings for him. After death of Ramesh, Baby stops her contact with the world and closes herself in her house. Before Kamal tries to kill Baby, Keshav friend of Ramesh helps Baby to get out the house and lead a happy life with him.

There are different layers of desire of Baby with all its complexity, memory of a family and knowledge that parents tried to kill her death of brother, feelings of love for her brother, relationship developed with Kamal. Amidst all this, the life in the house for Baby becomes torturous. It prompts her to close down all positive hopes in her life. There is always an entirely different world of experience for physically challenged people. It affects their every bit of consciousness. It changes everything about what they think about others and what they think that others think about them. Eventually it negatively affects their growth on every level. Her knowledge that her parents are responsible for her plight has very bad impact on her. It makes a world of difference when a person knows that someone else is responsible for lifelong deformity in one's body. Blame to nature and one's fate could be sometimes a factor offering certain type of strengths to such people. In case that of Baby who comes to know that her parents are responsible for her conditions has two levels of adverse effects i.e. her loss of object of desire in the form of father and mother and the void is filled with hatred and anguish for them.

Flower of Blood was first published in 1972. For Elkunchwar, this play was very important as we see from this play as he himself admits in an interview that there is no impact of western dramatic writings on it. With this play, he began to write plays which have images and thematic concerns which are woven in the fabric of story of the play most naturally and there are no conscious efforts on the part of the dramatist to bring in certain effects.

Flower of Blood does have a very disturbing situation. Bahu and Padma are husband and wife. Leelu and Shashi are their children. Shashi is killed in war. They have a paying guest Raja. Set in a very typical middle class family background, the play grows more complex with the complexity of desires on the part of the mother and the daughter when they have their own way of loving Raja. It grows disturbing and violent as the daughter does not understand her mother's motherly love for Raja and the mother does not understand the love feelings of Leelu for Raja. It is in this play also, Elkunchwar depicts his favourite thematic concern of futility and meaninglessness of human life.

It also becomes very clear that certain strong human traits tend to exploit the existing human relationships and in this 'play' of significance two possibilities become stronger i.e. complexities of existing relationships eventually resulting in conflicts of severe kind and realization of feeling of loneliness and denial of life. It is not always intelligible neither on the part of the characters nor on the part of any common human being to realize that the failure at coping up with the complexity of desire and understanding the nature of conflicts emerging out of the complexity, are the major reasons for the sorrows and pains felt by their minds. Loneliness, pain, helplessness and disinterestedness are the results of such complex culmination of desires. Venkat Murali Palla in his article entitled "Thematic Study of Mahesh Elkunchwar's Flower of Blood" talks about Padma's 'grasping of illusion' and says that:

> For Padma, Raja is the illusion which she tries to grasp. Sometimes, she looks upon him as her son and sometimes her sexual urge comes to the fore, she might have wanted him to a large extent as her sexual object in non-physical sense. She is unable to reconcile both, the maternal as well as sexual instincts, so she indulges in "Absurdio Reduction". The term reveals that though she argues illogically, she thinks that she is logical (Palla 227).

Elkunchwar seems to be stretching this level of complexity at a different level in his one act play *Kaifiyat* in the form of Rajeshwar's revenge on the world for its inability to understand him and his art. It results in brutal killing of his son Gopu by him. By and large, the play being the last one in the collection of his one acts entitled *Yatanaghar*, remains honest in exhibiting Elkunchwar's conscious attempt to present internal conflicts of humans on the stage. Process of creation and its complex nature are often sought by Elkunchwar as tools to present complexity of human existence. He becomes successful in showing how Rajeshwar has to lead life with meaningless and full of agony that people love and enjoy his art but fail to understand him as a person. The three women that become intimate part of his life also fail to understand him. It makes him realize the futility of his life and art. In fit of anger, he kills his son Gopu who is born out of his illicit relationship. The feelings of revenge on the world and destruction of artifacts dawn on him out of the sheer hopelessness and despair. Rajeshwar pleads for understanding his standpoint and views on why he did so. On his part, it is very painful to realize that none believes in him and supports him. He is given capital punishment.

Kaifiyat does have the elements that touch upon issues like absurdity, violence, revolt, desire and cruelty against backdrop of the question of conflict between world of reality in arts and reality of world.

Rudravarsha is another example of Elkuchwar's same line of thought. There are six characters in the play i.e. Rajiv, Jaya, Yashwant, Usha, Rajiv's mother and his family doctor. The relationship between husband and wife is the central theme of the play. However, the image of rain does imply the external factor's role in the plight of human beings and their submission. The complexity of desires and relationship among the two couples is driven by feelings of betrayal, underdeveloped growth of personality, inferiority complex and development of desire for a person other than one's partner.

What make the play with much variety of themes is love of doctor for his beloved who suffers from leprosy, the image of rain and strong optimism on the part of almost all characters. They otherwise become the integral part the centre i.e. husband and wife relationship between Rajiv and Jaya and Yashwant and Usha. Elkunchwar offers a fine depiction of state of desire between the husbands and wives and the doctor and his lover. Rajiv suffers from inferiority complex and his disturbed psyche is largely influenced and dominated by childhood memories of father who dominated and always looked down upon him for his constant failure. Due to the loss of confidence, he is not able to give satisfaction to his wife. The punctured psyche of

Rajiv constantly shadows his life with failures on various other fronts of life. His relationship with his wife as husband is main one. For Jaya, this fact is more complex. She loses her interest in him. There is lack of desire between the two.

For Yashwant, it had been a second marriage and he does family planning operation after the birth of the first child in his first marriage. He marries Usha after the death of his first wife. But he does not tell her that he has done such operation. When she comes to know about it, she feels deceived and lost. She loses desire for him. When Yashwant returns home after fourteen years, Usha spends time with Yashawant. She starts receiving satisfaction and solace in the company of Yashawant. *Rudravarsha* becomes Elkunchwar's one of the most significant plays that deals with man-woman relationship.

Garbo "an absurdist play ... thoroughly contemptuous of bourgeois pretensions" (Deshpande 31) perhaps is more explicit and vivid with sexuality, violence and obscenity among all plays of Elkunchwar. He himself admits that it was written with intention that he was a rebel in the field of creative writing. However he does not consider it a successful play on his level. He realizes that the artistic level of the play has degraded due to the lack of artistic representations. Intuc, Garbo, Pansy and Shrimant represent different sections in society. Though Elkunchwar does not rate the play as more serious, it does have thematic concerns that comment on issues like sexuality, violence and subjugation of women. The play very significantly deals with the three issues. Controversy was due to open depiction of the multiple sexual relations of Garbo with the three and others as well. She aborts the child and at the end Shrimant kills her and rest of the two are happy that she is dead.

The course of events and the dialogues of the characters reveal that arrival of new life is such a beautiful feeling and they are happy that Garbo is pregnant. She initially does not tell them the truth. She tells them it was an accident. But when they come to know that it was a conscious attempt by her to kill the child by opting for the scene in the film that included a camel ride. The dummy could have been used for the shot but she insisted on doing it herself and that resulted in the abortion. Though the play ends in murder of Garbo by the trio, it subtly values the world of reasons of the act by Garbo.

It shuns romantic ideas in society that bears a layer of void thought of sustainability in the long run. It lays bare the subjugation, plight and worsening conditions of women. The phenomenon of oppression of women is more complex than it appears. Lack of choice has been perhaps the main problem for women and they have to continue with atrocities and violence against them. The subjugation in case of Garbo is of multiple levels. Being a woman, being poor, being jobless, having no family and financial support and sacrifice of dreams that a common woman visualizes, have some of the levels. As a result, she kills the child but it eventually results in her death. Her death is also not grieved but rather justified by the three without understanding the conditions of Garbo. It is perhaps why Dr. Supriya Pendhari thinks that "the three had physical relations with Garbo only for satisfying their sexual desire. But when such desires are not satisfied by her, they kill her. They do not feel sad after her death because they love her only to satisfy their physical desires" (Pendhari 159). This desire also was one of the major concerns of the playwright as it is visible in the interview of Elkunchwar with Samik Bandyopadhyay. By referring to the interview, he writes about Garbo in the following way, in his introduction to the *Collected Plays of Mahesh Elkunchwar* Vol. I published by Oxford University Press.

> But as the 'filth' proliferates, with a series of exposures and confessions, Pansy charging Shrimant with

homosexual assault, Garbo takes responsibility for
corrupting Pansy ('Initially I played around with him
just for fun. Then it became a habit. An entertaining
game… I should have hardened my hearth at least
once. Pansy, you're still too young.), Shrimant
bringing his impotence out into the open, and Garbo
giving the true story of her abortion, the illusions
crash. (Bandyopadhyay xiv).

Unlike Pendhari, for Samik Bandyopadhyay, it is not
only the loss of object of desire (here it is both the child
and Garbo) for the three that instigates the murder but it is
the loss of hope for only possibility of their being satisfied,
the ability of creation of new life fulfilled and satisfaction
being potent. Dr. Sidney Shirly wrote an article for Journal
of English Lnaguage and Literature entitled "Sexuality
versus Psychology: A Study of Mahesh Elkunchwar's Garbo
and Desire in the Rocks". She analyses the functioning of
sexuality in Intuc, Shrimant and Pansy and says, "Sexuality
works in theses individuals as a mode of manifesting their
inner condition whether it is frustration or a desire to control.
The idea of sexuality is continuously evolving into various
complex meanings (Shirly 124). She quotes E Munck's idea
from his Ethics of Sexology who says that sexuality is no
longer governed by rigid religious rules and taboos today but
has become a very personal matter for the individual. This
observation by Munck is very apt to relate with the behavior
of the three male characters in the play.

Elkunchwar's penchant for the theme of artistic creation
and all aspects of process of creation is clearly visible in his
Desire in the Rocks. The two major characters i.e. Hemkant
and Lalita are brother and sister. They have sexual relation.
Hemkant is a sculptor and they have moved in a village where
they have their ancestral mansion. Hemkant has busied

himself in work of carving statues in the rocks around the village. Reasoning and uniformity of feelings that support the balance of mind of Lalita is sustained only till the time when she realizes that her brother does not love her truly. There was an understanding to Lalita that at a time it justified for her the incest relations of her with her brother. Memory plays an important role in the play on two event levels. The memory of Lalita of her house where she grew under the dominating authoritative regime of her father and loss of her mother has a vital role in the construction of her psyche. Hemkant for her is an only escape from the house. Her mind was so tormented that incest relationship was never to be negated by her. Another was the memory of the mansion where a beggar was buried under the basement of the mansion and a curse of the woman prevailed the mansion.

Lalita knows the taboo nature of their relationship. However, there was a strong uniformity within her mind as long as it was supported by the feelings that her brother loves her truly. The messing up of Hemkant in distinguishing between art and life results in shaking the fortification of Lalita's mind. And as a result, the whole burden of social obligations, cultural constraints and cynical responses from society built a wall of despair in front of Lalita. Such type of conditions, always leave an individual to clutch certain traditional religious views and seek solace in certain rituals and acts of renunciation. It even in case of Lalita goes to the level of self torture. As far as desire between the brother and sister is concerned, Lalita's revolt against the brother is concerned and violence in the form of suicidal end of their lives is concerned, the play offers a commentary on the thin line in human relationship that always does not hold on the 'fine balance'. There happens an event on psychological level of Lalita as about loss of object of desire and then the loss of cause of desire. Zizek recognizes the role of fantasy in construction and activation of desire. According to him fantasy realizes a desire in a systematic way or

> a fantasy constitutes our desire, provides its co-ordinates; that is, it literally 'teaches us how to desire'... fantasy meditates between the formal symbolic structure and the positivity of the objects we encounter in reality – that is to say, it provides a 'schema' according to which certain positive objects in reality can function as objects of desire, filling in the empty places opened up by the formal symbolic structure (Zizek 7).

It was a failure for Litata in the 'schema' which otherwise intact for a longer time. It is perhaps the same process in relation with negative object in reality that function as object of desire filling in the empty places opened up by the knowledge of futility, untruth and loss of cause of desire. Initially she loses the object of desire i.e. Hemkant and gradually the loss of cause of desire leads her to renunciation of everything that she had been holding close to her. It included her body as well. Dr. Sidney Shirly in her article "Sexuality versus Psychology: A Study of Mahesh Elkunchwar's Garbo and Desire in the Rocks" writes about the reason of frustration in the relation between the sister and brother in different manner. She says that "[t]he incomplete desires of Lalita and the objective passion of Hemkant result in their being frustrated. Incompleteness and barrenness enters their selves thereby punishing them from within" (Shirly 124).

Party is a quite different from the plays Elkunchwar wrote earlier. The play as far as the present research work is concerned has certain elements like revolt and violence that are used by the dramatist to suggest the workings of power and violent culmination of protest and movement against the power structures and its functioning. The party and incidents in it, offer us idea about various people and attitudes in society. For Neelam Man Singh *Party* is a play where "we see vignettes of Indian artistic life suffused with the politics of grants, trips, abroad and the tensions of manipulative power games" and according to her Elkuchwar in the play "takes a look at the members of the creative set in an Indian metropolis, with their pretentions, rivalries, aspirations, and frustration, even as they are stalked by the guilt of having betrayed one their own" (Singh 25). It is a party organized by Damayanti Rane at her house. It is organized in the honour of Barve for his achievement as an author. Many people related to the field of writing have gathered in the party. Elkunchwar succeeds in showing the hypocrisy of these party goers. Few members in the party represent fields like cinema, art and politics as well. The way the dramatist presents the course of events and the life and death of Amrit lays bare the difference between the people who live in society as so called social workers and the people who devote and sacrifice their lives for social cause.

A. Linda Primlyn in her article "The Sound of Silence in Mahesh Elkunchwar's Plays *Pond* and *Party*" calls *Party* as an expose of "Bombay's creative community where people live under false pretences subsiding their feelings. He tells that parties are false gaiety. Usually in parties people greet each other with wide smiles, and underneath their smiles there lies violence" (Primlyn 89). It is true that the structure of the play brings the climax with certain magnitude and leaves an impact on readers and audience. Death of Amrit proves an eye opener for all at the party. Amrit's selflessness, renunciation and positive attitude to work for the *adivasi* people, brings them idea how it is more important that Amrit life is worth valuing and it had more meaning than the lives they were living full of desires and vanity of false ambitions for fame and recognitions. Though the play seems to be an outcome of harsh responses on the part of the playwright to the hypocrisy of people especially from the middle class society, Ekunchwar does not rate this play as a systematic play in its structure. In his interview in 1996 with Anjum Katyal and Paramita Banerjee for *STQ*, he says, "I don't even rate it as a good play now. It's a clever play. I observed the people around me and I wrote it out. I didn't take any position in it, as a playwright" (Elkunchwar 9). There is a main reason behind this way of thinking of Elkunchwar and it is his reading and knowledge about the contemporary theatre and other writing. He compares it with the latest and most artistic writing. One thing must be made clear though Elkunchwar does not consider it a serious play that it has its major impact on readers and audience and relevance to contemporary politics at various levels.

Dnayneshwar Nadkarni in his review of *Party* points about certain 'lacks'. He writes, "Indeed the lack of 'dramatic' actions is the most serious flaw in this play. The many characters seem to float in limbo as literally they sail onto the three or four different sections of the acting area. There is … an attempt to present case studies … But there is very little novelty in what these case studies have to reveal to us" (Nadkarni 27).

Reflection by Elkunchwar falls in type of existential plays rather than absurd plays. It is a rich play with thematic concerns, representations, language, communication, structure and integrity. It is a very successful attempt on the part of the playwright to bring in novelty in structure and overall presentation. Like most of his other plays, there is minimization of characters as well. There is a widow, who is the owner of the house, a paying guest named Thokale, his friend Bawate and girl named Kersuni. Thokale is a clerk and one fine morning he stands in front of mirror and realizes that there is no reflection of him in the mirror. He is confused, perplexed and troubled by the discovery. He admits that his reflection is lost. The play subtly pictures the existential and identity crises in the life of middle class people. The widow tries to help Thokale as she has strong desire for him. Her actions clearly show the forces of desires she has bottled up within herself. Mr. Bawate also lost his reflection and instead he sees a reflection of a parrot in it. The fact that he lost his reflection, doe not trouble Bawate as much as it troubles the mind of Thokale. There is another character who lost her reflection and it is a girl Kersuni working in Thokale's office. She has loved Thokale secretly and as she realizes that Thokale too has lost his reflection, she identifies herself with him.

It is in this play, Elkunchwar has dealt with inevitable loss of identity of human beings. The technique Elkunchwar has deployed where these characters make attempts to enter each other's mind to find out their reflection forms a way out. However, the failure of the characters to find out their reflection makes the issue of loss graver. When Thokale commits suicide, the event also vanishes as if nothing has ever happened. It also becomes a commentary on today's interapersonal relationships and their irrelevance in the society.

It could also be related to the idea of Marx where he described alienated relationship of workers in the process of production. Such relationships in a stronger sense make the structures of society in the form of religion, institutions, idea of self, love, humanity void. It as we see it in many cases, degenerate the identity of individuals in their singularity. The inability of being effective in given structure and losing one's very base for such capability is disturbing at a very deep level of psyche. And there is every chance of having violent end to the actions and course of events. While writing review of Elkunchwar's plays like *Reflection* and *Autobiography*, Giridhar Rathi opines that

> [r]ealism, naturalism, surrealism, the absurd and such other modern trends have often taken a firm

grip over out playwrights. Mahesh Elkunchwar is a fine example of a sensitive mind keeping a watchful eye on the latest developments in the psychic human history. Very briefly put, the first one is a disturbing picture of middle-class ironies, while the second one unravels layers after layers of human volition, choice, compulsions and contradictions (Rathi 35).

It is true that for Elkunchwar middle class and its psychology, love for creation and its stimuli, human desires, effects on human psyche and relationships due to modernity and death, have been crucial issues. He seems to be at war with certainty and universality of the issues. His similar efforts could be seen very clearly as one categorizes his all plays in certain thematic structure. However, Beulah Rose in her article A Solution to the Question of Absurdity: Elkunchwar's *'Reflection'* thinks it an absurdist play. She writes that "[t]he vague background of the hero and his loss of identity all lead to emphasis one point – that Absurdity is a universal human condition. It cannot be circumscribed to one group or a particular region. It is the nameless … able to bring forth the terror and also a universal acceptability (Rose 27). Deepa Gahlot says that the term 'pratibimb' used by Elkunchwar for his play in Marathi meaning 'reflection' has multiple levels of meaning. She explores that it could be seen as a comedy as well. Besides it she says that it is thought provoking. While talking on the level of force, she says that "the play kicks in the absurdist tradition of raising existential questions. At the same time it warns you not to take it too seriously" (Quoted in Amrite 241).

In the play *Autobiography*, Rajadhyaksha a renowned writer living alone in his late seventies in his house and being interviewed by a young girl of twenty to twenty four named Pradnya. She is working on her project of assisting Rajadhyaksha in writing his autobiography. The life of the writer can be viewed through three perspectives one being the life of his own as an author who writes with certain responsibilities and moral values imbibed from nationalism and "the absolute morality that was intrinsic to Gandhi's political thought as well as its spiritual base" (Elkunchwar 115) particularly as an aftermath of struggle of independence and implementation of democracy in India and construction of a new nation. Secondly, the marital life of the writer with his wife Uttara does not prove to be happy as the couple is not able to beget a child of their own. And the appearance of Uttara's younger sister Vasanti in their family affects the life of the couple as Rajadhyaksha and Vasanti in the absence of Uttara get attracted to each other and the union result into the separation of the writer from the both the women. Thirdly, the solitude that is experienced by Rajadhyaksha after this break up, is majorly characterized by his realization nature of desire and his attempts to seek justification to it and ignorance about the fact that the child of Vasanti is his own.

Desire and revolt on the part of Vasanti has been a crucial part of the thematic concerns that affects life of both her sister Uttara and Rajahyaksha.

As One Discardeth Old Clothes... is perhaps one of the most important plays that reveal issue of desire which is so culture and time specific. It becomes an important document to register the function and nature of desire among the people even otherwise constrained by cultural regulations. The sway of desires is usually related with the cultural encroachment and modernism. The agents that affect strong actions instigated by desires at deeper level have effects externally caused by society, media, politics and visual productions of reality. They are rather different than the ones from within one's psyche and world of emotions.

The play has at least three levels of human experiences embedded in the life of traditionally fortified social structure of family and marriage institutions. In India, the institutions are the both guardians of Indian culture and values and also the main cause of sustenance of gender, social and economic discriminations. Aai's acts of extra-marital affairs suggest the possibilities of challenges a tormented woman can give. Elkunchwar chooses to deal with this aspect at the level of Aai's extra-marital affair and Baba's secret love for Kaku and vice versa. The three levels as mentioned earlier are set in Aai's act of affair, Baba's love for Kaku and Baba's obsession for Raghu and waiting for his death as he renounces everything and has no desire except for Raghu. Raghu remains a mystic figure throughout the play. At one level, it indicates a common experience as recounted by many people while being on deathbed. For Baba, it is a figure that he thinks has been there in his life and he could visualize him during certain incidents. The figure is nothing but his longings for a personality. It could be the desire of Baba for seeking solace in the company of the supernatural which could be a godly figure as the name suggests it. However, it could also mean as his alter ego that is visualized by him. It is a self that he always craved to live like.

Baba remains a central character in the play. As far as the structure of the play is concerned, Elkunchwar has woven a fine fabric of story, in which different characters that are the members of the same family, reveals their stories in way that keeps Baba in the centre. The authenticity of the play perhaps lies more in not only in the showing complexity of human experiences but in laying bare the invisible undercurrents in a culture, that otherwise would have been ideologically protected or neglected.

Wada Triology includes *Old Stone Mansion*, *Pond* and *Apocalypse*. *Old Stone Mansion* was published in 1982 after seven years of his writing *Party*. It is perhaps the best creation among his writings. Besides many other reasons, the depiction of life and culture in villages with all its poverty, fragmentation of family systems, regional disparities caused due to drought conditions. The play talks of more issues that are related to psychological orientations of people from the rural areas. The trilogy is much appreciated in Maharashtra and it had been quite successful on stage as well. Elkunchwar is known all over the world for the writing of these plays. There is also a line of critics who relate the structure and background of the play to the writing style that of Anton Chekov and his play *Cherry Orchard*. Kirti Jain registers that with writing of *Old Stone Mansion*, "[t]he rebellious writer seems to have grown up into a mature artist who now makes an epic sweep in recording the plight of a society in transition" (Jain 186).

Many critics have appreciated the trilogy and it has been major concentrations for the critics writing on Marathi plays in particular and Indian plays in general. As mentioned above, the trilogy holds significance on various levels that materializes certain untouched and abstract human experiences. Kirti Jain in her review list some of the levels as she says that the play *Old Stone Mansion* reminds her of Chekov's Cherry Orchard, "with its delicately etched characters, its ambience which itself is the meaning, and the subtle interplay between four generations as well as two worlds – those of the city and villages" (Jain 186). Jain rightly observes the scope of the thematic concern of the play though she connects it with that of Chekov's. Sudhanva Deshpande in his review of *Collected Plays of Mahesh Elkunchwar*, talks about Elkunchwar as a rebellious playwright and says that in *Old Stone Mansion*, Elkunchwar turns to the same 'realism' that he seemed 'loathe earlier'. He comments that "[w]ith a sensitive, almost anthropological gaze, he dissects the inner dynamics of a family that disintegrates as the village economy that sustained it hitherto crumbles" (Deshpande 31).

It is true that out of myriad aspects, the economic aspect that the play highlights is crucial one. It is the major issue that seems to be instigating and generating other responses through the character. At a certain level, they even shape and form emotional responses. Through the generations of Deshpande of Dharangaon, Elkunchwar has presented a complete picture of a family that unfortunately deteriorates and reaches to sad culmination. The trilogy does have the potentials that cross the boundaries of the experiences of certain Brahmin family and with the richness and commonness of the experience through generations, it remains applicable to many other families in Maharashtra. Perhaps it is the universality of experience that makes the play one of the most successful creations by Elkunchwar both on and off the stage. With the writing of *Pond* and *Apocalypse*, Elkunchwar succeeds in making it as an epic. As mentioned by Kirti Jain, Elkunchwar grows more mature and perhaps offers the best play to Marathi theatrical traditions. In his article *(Dis)locating Theoritical Catachresis in Mahesh Elkunchwar: A Playwrights Re-creative Journey from the Western Pages to the Practical World,* Sayan Dey relates the theme of the play with existential debate. He says that this work of Elkunchwar:

> Undertakes a steep journey into the rural chore exploring, investigating and evoking the multi-dimensional binaries of individual/clustered, eternal/external, male/female that has always been occupied the nucleus of post-modern existential debate. The Deshpandes of Dharangaon have been crippled by both geographical and economical aridity that has cruised into their life with the advent of post-independent progressive ethics of urbanization, modernization and industrialization (Dey, 287).

The play proved to be a milestone not only for the writing career of Elkunchwar. It also formed a major episode in whole Marathi tradition of playwriting. Chandrashekhar

Jahagirdar observes that the modernist tradition gave major playwrights and plays in sixties. But all of them seemed during seventies to reach a dead end by creating its stereotype. He considers that Elkunchwar and Shyam Manohar these two playwrights made a way out of 'frozen tradition of modernism'. He considers *Old Stone Mansion* as an important play for the use of very naturalistic tradition rejected by modernism. He further writes that *Old Stone Mansion* portrays tension in a joint family belonging to decadent aristocracy. For Prof. Jahagirdar the exploration "of love and conflict, emotional distance and proximity in familial relations, is so subtle and delicately powerful" (Jahagirdar 66) unlike others it reminds him one of Satyajit Ray's films *Shaka-Prashakha*.

Somnath Barure in his article "Mahesh Elkunchwar's *Old Stone Mansion* – End of an Ethos" talks about issues of 'influence' and 'borrowing' investigate the 'end of feudalism in India'. Like many other critics, Mr. Barure registers the all pervasiveness of cultural aspect in the play. He concludes his article saying that the ethos in the form of the fall of the age's long *wada* culture in India has "ill practices of not keeping pace with time that turned its enemy in Th future... The mansion seems to be caught into the mesh of tradition and modernity" (Barure 74). On the other hand the views of Nazneen Khan who rather didatively suggests Wada Trilogy as a form of Indian philosophy. The pervasiveness as suggested by Mr. Barure could be associated with the holistic idea proposed by Nazneen Khan in her article "Myriad Themes Immaculately Crafted in a Family Saga: Mahesh Elkunchwar's Wada Triology". She belives that the playwright through the trilogy "advises indirectly to seek one's origins, establish bonds with them, learn to look at one's suffering in a detached manner and prepare neself to be one with the larger entity. This is a philosophy... very close to the ancient Indian philosophy" (Khan 40). These speculations bring a very clear idea that the trilogy certainly is a literary forte of Elkunchwar. Madan Lal in his introduction to the second volume of *Collected Plays of Mahesh Elkunchwar* published by Oxford University Press writes about the differentiation between Elkunchwar's 'realism/naturalism on the one hand, and his absurdism/ symbolism on the other'. According to him these 'isms' "rests merely on the surface, for his philosophical concerns remain at heart the same, as we shall. As a director, I am much more intrigued stylistically by the potential pontency of puses and silences amidst his dialogue (Lal xxii). He goes on making very valuable observations that talk more meaningfully about Elkunchwar as a playwright and his literary productions. He says that there is "one strong cord unites all of Elkunhwar's drama: the individual's quest for fulfillment, or its social denial, with disillusionment waiting at every step of the way" (Lal xiii). He also recognizes a crucial trait of the art of the playwright that the individual in his plays is physically never alone. He populates his stage world with family or society and still the individual 'invariably feels lonely and it is also when he says that the 'empathy' does not come externally.

Works Cited

Adiga, Arvind. *The White Tiger*. New Delhi: Harper Collins, 2008. Print.

Amrite, Sandhya. *Elkunchwarachi Natyasrushti*. Napur: Vijay Prakashan, 1995. Print.

Bandyopadhyay, Samik. Introduction. *Collected Plays of Mahesh Elkunchwar Vol.I*. By Elkunchwar. New Delhi: 2009. Print.

Barure, Somnath. "Mahesh Elkunchwar's *Old Stone Mansion* – End of Ethos." *International Journal of English Language & Translation Studies*, 2:4 (2014):74. Web. 24 Oct, 2015.

Bhagat, Datta. "Marathi Natak: 1975 to 2000." *Marathi Natak Ani Rangbhumi*. ed. Shinde, Wishwanath and Smart, Himanshu. Pune: Pratima Prakashan, 2008. Print.

Bhagwat, Hemangi. "Dalit Theatre: A Theatre of Protest". *European Academic Research* 2:1 (2014): 384. Web. 11 Oct. 2015.

Chakroborty, Kaustav, ed. *Indian Drama in English*. New Delhi: PHI Learning Pvt. Ltd., 2011. Print.

Chattopadhyay, Malyaban. "A Historical Study of Ancient Indian Theatre – Communication in the Light of

Natyasastra". *Global Media Journal* 4:2 (2013): 12. Web. 3 Oct, 2015.

Deshpande, G.P., ed. *Modern Indian Drama: An Anthology.* New Delhi: Sahitya Akademi, 2000. Print.

Deshpande, Sudhnva. "The Radical Conservative." Rev. of *Collected Plays of Mahesh Elkunchwar*, 20.4. Sept.2010: 31. Print.

Dey, Sayan. "Contribution of Mahesh Elkunchwar in the Evolution of Post- Colonial Marathi Theatre: Tracing the Theatrical History". *International Journal of Humanities and Social Science Invention* 3:3 (2014): 18. Web.16 Aug, 2015.

Dey, Sayan. "(Dis)locating Theoritical Catachresis in Mahesh Elkunchwar: A Playwright's Re-creative Journey from the Western Pages to the Practical World." *International Journal of English Language, Literature and Humanities* 2:10 (2015):287. Web. 16, Oct, 2015.

Elkunchwar, Mahesh. *Collected Plays of Mahesh Elkunchwar Vol. I.* New Delhi: Oxford University Press, 2009. Print.

Elkunchwar, Mahesh. *Collected Plays of Mahesh Elkunchwar Vol. II.* New Delhi: Oxford University Press, 2011. Print.

Elkunchwar, Mahesh and Anjum Katyal. "A Playwright of Human Relationships: An Interview with Mahesh Elkunchwar." *Seagull Theatre Quarterly* 22 (1999): 9. Print.

Goodman, Randolph. *Drama: A View from the Wings.* New York: Rinehart & Wilson, 1978. Print.

Jain, Kirti. "Chronicles of a Disturbing Time." Rev. of *Collected Plays of Satish Alekar: Collected Plays of Mahesh Elkunchwar, The Little Magazine*, 8.1 June, 2009: 186. Print.

Jahagirdar, Chandrashekhar. "Marathi Drama After 1960." *Haritham* 5 (1995):66. Print.

Khan, Nazneen. "Myriad Themes Immaculately Crafted in a Family Saga: Mahesh Elkunchwar's *Wada Trilogy.*" *The Quest,* 28:1 2014): 40. Print.

Khandagale, M. H. "A Short Survey of Contemporary Indian Drama." *Reflection of the Changing Indian Society in Indian English Drama.* ed. Bedre, R. T & Kadam. S. N. Narwadi: New Man Publication, 2013. Print.

Kulkarni, Purnima. "Subalterns Speak in Mahesh Elkunchwar's *Holi".* *Contemporary Discourse* 6:1 (2015): 219. Web. 20 Oct, 2015.

Lal, Madan. Introduction. *Collected Plays of Mahesh Elkunchwar Vol. II,* By Elkunchwar. New Delhi: (2011): xxii. Print.

Leader, Darian and Judy Groves. *Introducing Lacan, Duxford: Icon Books, 2000. Print.*

Mehta, Vijaya. Foreword. *Collected Plays of Mahesh Elkunchwar Vol. I,* By Elkunchwar. New Delhi: 2011. Print.

Mohan, Indra T.M.J.. "Post – Colonial Writing – Trends in English Drama". *The Indian Review of World Literature in English* 2:2 (2006): 5. Web.2 Jan, 2015.

Nadkarni, Dnyaneshwar. "Elkunchwar's 'Party'." *Enact,* (1976): 27. Print.

Palla, Venkat Murali. "Thematic Study of Mahesh Elkunchwar's *Flower of Blood".* *International Journal of Multidisciplinary Educational Research* 3:7 (2014) 227. Web. 19 Oct, 2015.

Pendhari, Supriya. *Marathi Natyasrushtitil Vidroh ani Navata.* Nagpur: Vijay Prakashan,2002. Print.

Primlyn, A. Linda. "The Sound of Silence in Mahesh Elkunchwar's Plays: *The Pond* and *Party".* *The Atalantic Literary Review Quarterly* 14:3 (2013): 89. Print.

Rathi, Giridhar. "The Indian Crucible." Rev. of *Pratibimb Aur Aatmakathaa. The Book Review,* 20.4 Nov, 1996: 35. Print.

Rose, Beulah. "A Solution to the Question of Absurdity in Elkunchwar's *'Reflection'." The Quest* 8:2 Feb, 1994: 27. Print.

Thokor, Daxa. "Social Issues in *Where There's a Will".* *Galaxy: International Multidisciplinary Research Journal* 1:1 (2012): 2. Web. 10 Jan, 2015.

Shirly, Sidney. "Sexuality Versus Psychology: A Study of Mahesh Elkunchwar's *Garbo* and *Desire in the Rocks*". *Journal of English Language and Literature 2:1*(2015): 124. Web. 12 Oct, 2015. Print.

Singh, Neelam Man. "Spearheading Modernism." Rev. of *Collected Plays of Mahesh Elkunchwar* Vol.II, The Book Review 36.12. Dec, 2012: 25. Print.

Zizek, Slavoj. *The Plague of Fantasies.* London: Verso, 1997. Print.

Chapter **II**

'DESIRE' IN THE SELECT PLAYS
OF MAHESH ELKUNCHWAR

Mahesh Elkunchwar seems to be mainly influenced by a certain philosophical thinking about the presentation of human nature on the stage. Death, sexuality, absurdity and vanity of human wishes are some of the most prominent themes that he pays more attention to. Desire formulates the core of almost every animate thing on the planet. Elkunchwar's presentation of desire on the stage exhibits certain traits. He brings about the representation of desire in certain ways in which it could best be expressed and secondly it is a learning process on the part of the playwright to understand the nature of the human relationship. It could be difficult to register how certain influences affect the style of one's writing. It is almost impossible to trace totality of impact on Elkunchwar's writings.

Elkunchwar's initial writing inspiration could be related to the writing style of the playwrights like Anton Chekhov and Vijay Tendulkar. Impressionism, existentialism and absurdity remain the characteristics of his plays as far as the plays that depict desire in man-woman relationship. Such plays oddly may include *Garbo, Desire in the Rocks, Autobiography, Flower of Blood, Party, Holi, As One Discardeth Old Clothes* ..., and *Reflection.* However they represent ethos that could be identified as the true picture of Indian culture. Writers like Satish Alekar and Vijay Tendulkar attempted depiction of desire in their plays and succeeded in making the groundbreaking revelations of Indian culture. Their plays like *Sakharam Binder, Vultures, Ghashiram Kotwal, Baby, Silence! The Court is in Session, Deluge, Begum Barve,* are some of the plays that deal with the theme. The main difference that lies among the each writer's writing is the spacio-temporal conditions that prevail the general writings along with the other contributing factors.

There are two ways of approaching the theme of desire in literature. One can take the moments of desire and analyze its connection with the immediate factors that influence and instigate it along with their contexts and their connection with psychological orientations. Secondly one can probe into the issue of desire finding out its broader sociological, political and economical perspectives originating from certain ideological constructions. This chapter attempts to evaluate the issue of desire in both the ways.

The word 'desire' is frequently taken and understood in the manner implying sexual orientation. It is a common practice. However the word is also used in everyday life situation meaning as 'longing' for something. Its use usually changes according to its object. If the object is material, it tends to mean a wish or longing to have or possess it but in case of person as the object of the verb, it means longing for someone that could be predominantly 'sexual'. While talking about the definition of the word we find that in the volume III of *The Oxford English Dictionary*, the word 'desire' is defined as "to long for (something lost); to feel loss of, miss, regret, desiderate" and "to have a strong wish for; to long for, covet, crave." (247) In the 8th edition of *Oxford Advanced Learner's Dictionary*, the word desire is defined as "(--for sth) a strong wish to have or do sth" and "(--for sb) a strong wish to have sex with sb." (Turnbull 411) The dictionary gives the meaning of the word as a verb as "to want sth; to wish for sth" and "to be sexually attracted to sb". (411). This predominant connection of the meaning of word desire with sexuality suggests the vital role of sexuality or sexual desire in human life.

In his documentary entitled *Pervert's Guide to Cinema*, Slovej Zizek attempts the evaluation of the sexuality in the movies like *Birds, Psycho, etc* by Hitchcock in light of Lacanian psychoanalyses and Neo Marxist ideology. He announces, "There is nothing spontaneous about our desire… We are taught to desire" (Zizek). This sets a broader context for us to evaluate the motivations behind the seemingly natural phenomenon called human instincts. It leads us to critically analyze how in a social context certain relations are labeled as 'queer' and 'natural' whereas the phenomenon if considered a result of particular social order and formalized and accepted social inter and intra personal relations, it becomes essential to trace the mechanism of the instinct and the artificiality of its origin and structure. It also becomes essential to identify the true conditions related with origin of desires and the portion of external social agents in it.

Kamasutra, a canonical text on sexuality was produced in India. The text was compiled by Vatsyayana during the 4th century AD. It is translated by Sir Richard Francis Burton (1821-90) who was a British explorer and the translator of *One Thousand and One Nights.* Vatsyayana defines *Kama* as

> the enjoyment of appropriate objects by the five senses
> of hearing, feeling, seeing, tasting and smelling,

assisted by the mind together with the soul. The ingredient in this is a peculiar contact between the organ of sense and its object, and the consciousness of pleasure that arises from that contact is called Kama. Kama is to be learned from the *Kamasutra* (aphorisms on love) and the practice of citizens (Burton 02).

There are various issues that are essential to be considered while studying the conditions in which the text *Kamasutra* was produced. The most important of them was that it was written for the members of king's family in particular and common citizen in general. The text offers the practical analyses of sexual performances with all its details where sexual gratification of the partner is valued the most. The references that he makes about the sexuality as a weapon to use against the enemies suggests its vital monarchial orientations. There are many factors Vatsyayana deals with detailing their sex wise psychological and physiological differences.

Auddalika in the same treatise says that females do not emit as males do. The males simply remove their desire, while the females, from their consciousness of desire, feel a certain kind of pleasure, which gives them satisfaction, but it is impossible for them to tell you what kind of pleasure they feel. The fact from which this becomes evident is that males, when engaged in coition, cease of themselves after emission, and are satisfied, but it is not so with females. She asks Vatsyayana the need of different work on the part of male and female when the semen of female fall in the same way as that of male. He replies:

> ...this is also so because the ways of working, as well as the consciousness of pleasure in men and women, are different. The difference in the ways of working, by which men are the actors and women are the persons acted upon, and vice versa. And from this difference

in the ways of working follows the difference in the consciousness of pleasure, for a man thinks, 'This woman is united with me', and a woman thinks, 'I am united with this man' (Burton 17).

The contribution of Vatsyayana becomes significant due to main reason that he identifies the importance of peculiarity of orientation of female sexuality. His is the positive attitude towards the female sex and insists on importance of learning the art of love by the both male and female. It represents the period in Indian history when women were considered worthy of learning though he believed that the learning of *Kamasutra* should be continued "along with its arts and sciences, before marriage, and after it they should continue to do so with the consent of their husbands" (Burton 3).

The result of ideological forces of patriarchy very systematically ignored the presence of difference of female sexuality. The gradual subjugation of women resulted in erasing the identity of female sexuality. Until recently there was the manifesto of feminist movements that give call for necessity of realization of female as different, independent person. Vatsyayana however does not offer any remark on the issue of authenticity and artificiality of sexuality which mainly is considered as the territory of males to enjoy. It is why the back cover of the book *Kamasutra* reads that it as an indisputable classic of world literature, the *Kamasutra* remains one of the most enjoyable texts of antiquity. A work of philosophy, psychology, sociology, Hindu dogma, scientific inquiry and sexology, it has, at the same time, both affected Indian civilization and remained an indispensable key to the understanding of it.

However there remains a question that the openness that could be seen in the treatise of Vatsyayana could never become the part of such books in India until recently and the issue became taboo as a result of fortification of social institutions.

Foucault attempts to trace such similar development in relation with the European literature and expression of sexuality. In the beginning of *The History of Sexuality: An Introduction* Foucault writes how "certain frankness was still common… Sexual practices had little need to secrecy; words were said without undue reticence, and things were done without too much concealment; one had a tolerant familiarity with the illicit" (Foucault 03). But Victorian regime carefully confined sexuality and never allowed bodies to have "display of themselves".

It is most probably the second part of nineteenth century when the impact of Renaissance had been causing changes in Europe and England. It became a source of the change for India as Indian scholars receiving education from the country initially were influenced by the scientific ideas and felt a need of social and religious changes. It resulted in abolition of practices like *sati* and encouraging widow marriages. India had to see twentieth century for the woman to write a book like *Stri-Purush Tulana* by Tarabai Shinde or Maharshi Dhondo Keshav Karve to marry a widow. The role played by ideology in making the sexuality a taboo resulted negatively especially in the context of women who for ages suffered from the evils of patriarchy. Since the Vedic period in India, there had been many customs and traditions that were followed without any interrogation. Silence on the issue of sexuality was one of them. Those became the target of conservatism, who tried to violate the silence.

In case of *Charvak* in Vedic period of India, silence, subjugation, prohibition and violence took place against them as the result of Vedic principles and their followers could not bear the thought of denial of God and reason as superior to Vedas. Dr. A.H. Salunkhe mentions in his book *Astikshromani Charvak* that one of the *Charvaks* who followed *Charvakdarshan* was killed and the incident is described in the

Mahabharat by one of the followers of Vedas. *Charvaks* were the followers of a set of beliefs according to which nothing could surpass the clear stream of reasoning in living a life and there existed no God. Foucault observes a similar thing about the classical age. He says,

> We are informed that if repression has indeed been the fundamental link between power, knowledge, and sexuality since the classical age, it stands to reason that we will not be able to free ourselves from it except at a considerable cost: nothing less than a transgression of laws, a lifting of prohibitions, an irruption of speech, are instating of pleasure within reality, and a whole new economy in the mechanisms of power will be required. For the least glimmer of truth is conditioned by politics (Foucault 5).

Perhaps, it is the cost mentioned by Foucault *Charvaks* had to pay. Along with the other revolutionary ideas of *Charvaks*, their ideas of *kama* were repressed. They were condemned to prohibition, nonexistence, and silence. It was not only that every possible kind of pleasure from sex was denied but also the 'knowledge to be gained from sex and the right to speak about it' was denied. Dr Salunkhe says that *Charvaks* propagated ideas of freedom to women about sexual expression. The ideas were realistic, rational and based on empiricism. As they posed direct opposition to Vedic ideology, they had been reduced to the nonexistent status. Vedic followers rigorously maintained the silence and *Charvaks* were perfectly labeled as atheists. The labeling made them anti-religious and in the course of time the sect remained in the minds of few people only as a notorious, hedonistic sect and for most of the other it was non-existent entity.

Foucault's idea is that sexuality is not an innate or natural quality of the body but rather the effect of historically specific power relations, falls in the thought line similar to that of Zizek or vice versa. According of Foucault science helped to create a sexual and social order that organizes and regulates ones' bodies, desires and identities and social behaviors. Foucault articulates this perspective. He reminds that silence itself is the integral part of power relations.

> Silence itself the things one declines to say or is forbidden to name...is less the absolute limit of discourse. The other side from which it is separated by a strict boundary, than an element that functions alongside the things said with them and in relation to them within strategies -There is no binary division to be made between what one says and what one cannot say...There are not one but many silences, and they are integral part of strategies that underlie and permeate discourses (Quoted in Narrain 27).

For Foucault, resistance is never in a position of exteriority in relation to power. According to him, the regulatory powers of literary discourses, psychiatry and jurisprudence which acted upon 'perversity' made the possibility of reverse discourses. Homosexuality began to speak on its own behalf to demand that its legitimacy or "naturality" be acknowledged often in the same vocabulary using same categories by which it to medically disqualified (Foucault 101).

After this realization, it is clear that the word desire necessarily carry the aura of meaning of sexual attraction combined with the presence of the factors like ideology, social norms, religion and so on. In work of criticism of the select plays of Elkunchwar, desire has been taken as an object of the study. The desire aimed is taken in those contexts when it appears to make its vital impact on the life of the characters or the course of the story of the plays like *Desire in the Rocks,*

Flower of Blood, Garbo, Autobiography, Reflection, Holi, As One Descardeth the Clothes… and *Yatanaghar.* The desires depicted are taken for consideration in the course of analyses to unfold the whole network of stimulus and response in human relationships and the very basis of its existence.

The last part of the twentieth century was the time when Elkunchwar wrote the plays like *Desire in the Rocks* and *Garbo.* Though his treatment of the issue in his writings is manifold, sexual desire's depiction is path breaking in the plays. The plays were controversial as they appeared on the scene of Indian Marathi commercial theatre and caused much upheaval at literary and political circles. Embodying dramatic form to the themes like incest and prostitution was not an inviting practice at the time of their arrival. Consequently they had to face strong opposition. This fact suggests the strength of the social practice of keeping silence on forbidden issues and subjects.

The culmination of the desires in the plays brings about whole problematic of human relationships. They characteristically receive violent, unpleasant and negative end. This kind of end could be observed frequently. Lalita and Hemkant in *Desire in the Rocks* embraces 'death by fire' as the *wada* is set on fire by the village people. Garbo in *Garbo* is killed by lusty and disappointed people like Shrimant, Pansy and Intuc. In *Autobiography* Anant Rajadhyaksha, Pradnya, Uttara and Vasanti have a complex network of relationship that ultimately reveals that human desires are not so easy to analyze though they may have simple appearance. In *Flower of Blood* the daughter and mother confront with each other at war whose reason and nature of motivation are different. Feeling of love of the young daughter, and feelings of love of the mother who lost her son and vainly attempts to seek the redemption of the loss of it in Raja, get complexly mixed and result into conflict.

Elkunchwar's writing has variety of desires that describe human relationships in their specifications, unique qualities and strangeness. His *Desire in the Rocks, Garbo, Reflection, Autobiography* and *Flower of Blood* present the problematic of taboo relations like incest, prostitution, unfulfilled desires, motivated desires and desires that human mind seeks in order to gain substitute for the loss it has experienced.

Elkunchwar subtly describes the complex part of the Indian society in its wake of modernity. It was intentional on the part of the author to treat the subject and lay bare the complications that have been concealed and presentation of Indian life always sought as uniform, having solid bondage and renunciation of pleasure principle. However this presentation by the author marks an outstanding beginning of a style of writing that went on becoming most effective and intense on various levels. Treatment to the issues like incest and prostitution could be very daring at the time when the author wrote it in the 1980s.

It was the period of great social change exactly before Indian independence. There has hardly a time when sexual desire was discussed and exhibited in any form of literature until the wave that dominated the writing of few Indian poets, novelists and playwrights. Mohan Rakesh's *Halfway House* and *Sakharam Binder* by Vijay Tendulkar are some of the instances. Foucault's mention about the 'certain frankness' about expression of sexual practice being common during seventeenth century has a British context. In Indian context, it has been largely different due to the strict and dominating religious ideas about giving priority to soul rather than body. The silence mentioned by Foucault is more prominent in this context and it hailed from the ancient times.

Elkunchwar's attempt to write *Garbo* could be viewed as resistance to silence maintained by various means. It was however not only the intention as he admitted to be about writing a play to shake and shock the minds of Marathi people of the time but it has also been an expression of the sexual practices in the parts of society that existed against the regime of the power that maintained the silence about the sexuality and carefully sought the nonexistence of such practices from the eyes of common people denying it every kind of appearance in formal society. Interestingly it is still maintained in the minds of common Indians and discovery of such practices is labeled either illegal or obscene. The attempts of Elkunchwar to write about such desires, however does not limit only to expression of the issue with certain frankness but also it is an of its existence with certain aura of importance of the issue in itself and its significance in relation to the other issues of human life from social and psychological perspectives.

Garbo has four characters through whom Elkunchwar presents the innermost spaces of consciousness of Indian society. Shrimant, Pansy, Intuc and Garbo represent psychological and social segments of society at the same time. Their names also clearly suggest the intention of their creation. Shrimant represents the haves possessing legitimacy to enjoy every kind of pleasure their fancy desires and Garbo represents garbage hence full of desire. Intuc is the intellectual strata of society that thinks itself equipped with the weapon called knowledge with the help of which they distinguish between what is good and what is bad for society ultimately conceiving themselves as the judges. Pansy is that immature psyche of any society largely driven by fancy and tends to act on superficial level.

They also represent various stages of totality of experiences in life of a human being. Emotions play an important role in our life and childhood, teenage, adulthood, old age, etc. are predominantly governed by certain emotions. Those segments of life undergo the benefits and disadvantages of their own. Simultaneously qualitative characteristics of the three exhibit the longing for status and privilege enjoyed by the other. Pansy craved for richness possessed by Shrimant. Shrimant on the other hand could not bear the thought of living alone without his friends. This contrast in desire however is governed by absurdist thinking towards futility of life.

Shrimant is predominantly driven by sexual desires and Intuc tells Pansy what Shrimant said about organizing a music concert,

> I once said to him, come on, cough up a thousand chips for some really good music. So he says, I hope she's going to be a female. So I said, 'Done. A female it shall be.' So the bastard says, 'What are her tits like?' that was the end of that little plan (Elkunchwar 14).

Shrimant believes he could buy every kind of happiness but is tormented by the feeling of unavailability of such pleasure and says, "A whole morning wasted. Didn't meet a soul. Those girls need bring down a peg or two. Shrin wasn't home. Babi said, 'I'm indisposed!' to hell with you. And there's still the entire day to get through. I hope at least Garbo turns up..." (Elkunchwar 12) But internally he is afraid of losing the company of his friend and thus horrified by the thought of being left alone whereas Pansy does not like the talk of Intuc but he can never tolerate the silence. He tells Intuc that he should keep talking as it gives a feeling of comfort to Pansy. The silence of Intuc for Pansy is scary. He begs Intuc to say something. And he mentions that the arrival of Shrimant would bring him certain entertainment to pass time pleasantly.

Pansy always craves for being rich like Shrimant though his is the life that seems to be moving to and fro between the values Shrimant and Intuc represent. Intuc who considered himself an intellectual also admits that the concepts of fame and popularity in life are a void. When asked about greatness by Pansy he replies,

I thought so at first. And then suddenly I felt disgusted. And this talk of fame is utter crap! People are fools… Fame is a sort of nonsense. Forget about whole thing and wallow happily in boredom. People are worse frauds than you think… All they want is somebody's boots to lick (7-8).

The trio has a peculiar relationship with Garbo who is "prepared to bed with anybody who'll give (her) a role" (38). Shrimat call her 'a sex machine' and says she is great in bed. The responses of the trio to the desires for Garbo are driven by specific orientations that are in a way result of the social, economic factors that have been responsible in constructing their psyche. For Shrimant she is a sex machine, for Intuc the relation with her is 'sacred and sublime' and for Pansy it is a 'rare and beautiful experience'. Intuc says that it doesn't make any difference if they call Garbo by different names as she would remain Garbo, while they will continue to search for the kind of Garbo they want. He confesses that in this process if they find Garbo that they wanted to find, it will be a good thing. But if they fail to find her in the certain form, suffering becomes inevitable. And while insisting on letting Garbo to be what she is, Intuc emphasizes that they should first know what they themselves really are. According to him, this would be a 'sound enough basis for their relationships with her'. The following is the remark by Intuc that could be called as an underlined thought as far as discourse on sexual desires is concerned. According to Intuc all the business about woman being an enigma and all that is a myth. He calls it a bit of literary truth. He contributes to man-woman relationship saying once one understands a woman; one does not want to look at her again. He adds that once one explores her, the thrill is gone. Here 'explore' has more significance of 'sex'. Intuc's philosophy about women takes an ultimate turn when he comments rather gender biasedly that a woman should be able to satisfy you fully, and yet withhold a part of her from you.

As it gets unbearable to Garbo to listen to the talk of Shrimant and Intuc, she starts to go out and Pansy begs her to stay there. It is here Intuc tells that it is her escape as he has his 'morbidity', Shrimant has 'perversity' and she has her 'sentimentality'. It is here she according to Shrimant, is more sentimental but he fails to recognize that it had been difficult all along for her to bear the nonsensical talk from the trio ever after her telling that she is pregnant. The thought of abortion is not comforting her. As the pressure builds upon her about thinking positively to give birth to the child, she breaks down and opens up saying she wants to love somebody one day and lose herself in love. But also realizes the impossibility of it. When she says that under hopeful desires lies a burning coal, it suggests that she has completely realized any positivity of thought will not work for her. And major cause of trouble comes from within her. She understands it in the form of being unable to live it up with the same intensity.

After the role play, Garbo frequently mentions how dirty and filthy lives they are living. This thought has been the result of her understanding that her pregnancy had been against the impossibility of a relationship that would never find a place in legitimacy of social norms. The feelings of disgust do not dawn upon only Garbo but all of them. Intuc also says that the conditions make you feel revolted. He tells that it is not the matter that only they are living such bad conditions but everywhere there is filth. He finds no clean place there. For the wallowing in filth means there is no escape from it; it is inevitable. It is here he tells the human reality that one live under certain conditions and one has oppositions to the conditions. However it culminates into accepting the situation and bringing out positivity of thought about the conditions. He says that in order to render the filth endurable, we will have to make up new theories about beauty. It could be a sort of aesthetics of filth and depravity.

At the end of the act first, Intuc insists Garbo on giving up the idea of hers about abortion. Initially Intuc grows very uncomfortable and is afraid that Garbo would blame them and they had to take the responsibility. He also insists her to accept money from Shrimant but she rejects it. Realizing his mistake, he starts pleading her to give birth to the child. Shrimant and Pansy also join him. Thought of bringing up the child pleases them and the news that Garbo is pregnant brings them a meaningful reason for their existence and they dream of the beautiful creation that could be a way to retain the guarantee of their perpetuation of their kind. Beautified and glorified idea of motherhood is not appreciated by Garbo. She realizes the difficulty of sustaining the life against the danger of losing her livelihood due to the pregnancy and impossibility of receiving the name of father for the child. She knows the idea of bringing the child in the world means making the child face the crude realities of social life even before it is mature enough to understand the concept of society itself. Intuc is full of romantic ideas about the phenomenon called creation. He says,

> What an awesome thought, that we are the cause for the birth of something beautiful… You are life about to give to another life…I wonder what the earth feels when a sapling takes root, grows, and blossoms. To give birth to a life, a living, breathing bit of blood and bones which grows… he will be like… a messenger from the gods, who will wander around the world embracing its sorrows (Elkunchwar 44).

The reaction of the trio to the news that the child was aborted and that was an accident, was that of loss and care for

Garbo. It was the desire to own the feeling of being a father. Though the desire stems from different sources within the individuals, it is the unique thing that unifies them to the core and each one of them insist her to go with him to live her rest of her life. It was in Garbo the three of them received the origin of a life that could bring them a solace from the penance of loss, lack of satisfaction in life and a void created from the feeling of impotency. Shrimant finds the roots of the cause in money. He expresses his wish for renunciation of wealth. He realizes that money is the root of all that happened. He recalls how from his teenage he had been used to worldly pleasures of body. He wanted at the time only 'things of flesh'. For Shrimant the child was the only hope to give him a label of becoming father though it was not real either. And the only chance was lost. It was a helpless effort on the part of Shrimant to sustain his name through the child. The birth of the child would have formed a meaningful whole in his life which is full of sexual despairs. He exploited all the possibilities of sexual pleasure and lost everything in the pursuit of those pleasures. The loss of child was the loss of object of desire for him. The positivity of it would have functioned as filling of gaps formed by the impotency he has developed.

For Intuc the child was the only way to get rid of the vicious impossibilities of the world and it could bring him a feeling of completeness in the form of happiness of a creation. It was the reason he always told Garbo how she is lucky to possess the happiness and potentials of creation and ability to give birth to an entirely new life. The death of the child was a return to 'filth'. He says, "The world we desired was not for us, could never have been. We were idiots, out to turn dreams into reality. Let's go back to our old world now. The world of filth. As a punishment. And as a sort of consolation too" (49).

Intuc suffers from the anguish that he has lost beauty; the ability to create and everything worth possessing. According to him, he is at war with beauty and 'the very concept it represents'. Beauty remains only 'a figment of imagination, 'a sort of mirage', and á trap'. The feeling of loss makes him think that 'filth is the only truth' and it is the only choice they are left with. He determines to choose it and live with it. He feels a strange freedom now and feels a strange numbness 'without experiencing any emotion'. It is with the despair of desire, three are devasted. It is why Dr. Sidney Shirly in her paper "Sexuality versus Psychology: A Study of Mahesh Elkunchwar's Garbo and Desire in the Rocks" writes that "[s] exuality works in these individuals as a mode of manifesting their inner condition whether it is frustration or a desire to control. The idea of sexuality is continuously evolving into various complex meaning" (Shirly 124). She thinks that the three characters along with Garbo meet a destructive end and sexuality in an uncontrolled, savage atmosphere is the major reason.

As far as the structure of the play *Garbo* is concerned, Chandrashekhar Jahagirdar does not rate it a systematic play. He writes in his article entitled "Marathi Drama after 1960" that the playwright could not always find a perfect correlation between modernist experimental techniques and the thematic compulsions of the text. The treatment of sexuality in the plays like *Desire in the Rocks* and *Garbo* is "a kind of modernist experiment which, being too loud, rhetorical and self-conscious is somewhat detrimental to the themes... These are some of the sad examples of the ideological gap between technique and text" (Jahagirdar 64).

In the play *Autobiography*, Rajadhyaksha a renowned writer is living alone in his late seventies in his house and being interviewed by a young girl of twenty to twenty four named Pradnya. She is working on her project of assisting Rajadhyaksha in writing his autobiography. The life of the writer can be viewed through three perspectives; one being the life of his own as an author who writes with certain responsibilities and moral values imbibed from nationalism and "the absolute morality that was intrinsic to Gandhi's political thought as well as its spiritual base" (115) particularly as an aftermath of struggle of independence and implementation of democracy in India and construction of a new nation. Secondly, the marital life of the writer with his wife Uttara does not prove to be happy as the couple is not able to beget a child of their own. And the appearance of Uttara's younger sister Vasanti in their family affects the life of the couple as Rajadhyaksha and Vasanti in the absence of Uttara get attracted to each other and the union result into the separation of the writer from the both the women. Thirdly, the solitude that is experienced by Rajadhyaksha after this break up, is majorly characterized by his realization of nature of desire and his attempts to seek justification to it and ignorance about the fact that the child of Vasanti is his own.

The desire begotten against this background brought the feeling of being wronged to the both Rajadhyaksha and Vasanti. Though Vasanti admits that it is mainly the patronizing gesture of Uttara that prompted her revenge and she decided to win against Uttara since the insult caused by Uttara piled up. Vasanti tells Uttara that she could not bear her arrogance. It refuses to even raise an eyelid and glance at anyone else. She tells Uttara that she was so immersed in herself, smugly feeding on her inflated ego.

Desires indeed have various ingredients that are composed of different set of situations, cultures, psyches, ways of seeing, ideas of satisfaction and morality, absence and presence and so on. The desire in the context of this play originates perhaps seemingly very trivial cause as compared to the desires depicted in *Desire in the Rocks, Garbo, Flower of Blood* and *Yatanaghar*. They are antagonistic feelings of a woman for her sister who treats her very badly. It was the same woman who treated her so lovingly when she was a kid and both of them were staying with their parents. But as she got married to Rajadhyaksha, she changed completely. The feelings of arrogance, vanity and egotism quickly took over her and she started behaving badly with parents as well as with her younger sister. As a result of it, Vasanti says to Uttara, "I dint ever want to compete with you. But when you began to assume the pose of a patron, I decided … I'd defeat you.. by taking away that one thing that gave you all your sense of power" (143).

The complexity of the desire affected the trio so deeply that the aftermath of it resulted in spending rest of their lives in separation from their 'love'. Sexual desire of Rajadhyaksha for Vasanti caused a great deal of pain to Uttara for she could not bear the thought her husband going close to someone physically. In turn, the act suggests and provides her with set of other feelings.

On a common ground level, it is the feeling of love that one enjoys possessing and being possessed. Marriage offers the possibility and in a way guarantee for such a possession. The dispossession of it causes whole universe of problematic for the both husband and wife. Presence of sexual desire for someone else other than the partner brings about the feelings of loss of emotional support on certain levels. This loss however proves to be the most important factor in the separation of partners in a marriage. The act does not only bring the feeling of void of disappearance of emotional support that has been always felt and taken for granted for its longevity of existence till the end of life but it also challenges one potentials and ability being capable of possessing certain things like love and it is the thing that forms core of human life in love relationship. It is the loss of the feeling of being able to be capable of bringing sexual gratification and happiness to someone. A member of a couple could never conceive the possibility of sexual gratification of the other member in his/her absence and realization of such act brings again the feeling of loss of the unique feature that his/ her mind perceived and imagined about. It is monopoly one enjoys worth possessing. And the loss of this monopoly closes the possibility of restructuring the relationship again. Even attempted, the presence of the image of the act brings forth the impossibility of such construction and it produces the feeling of hatred and outrage in the mind of the person. Revenge is a common experience in such cases. Violence is seen more often at this point of time. Violent acts are more frequent when the male partner is wronged.

Alix Kats Shulman in her article "Sex and Power: Sexual Bases of Radical Feminism" mentions the history of British feminism and how sexuality was confined to certain institutions and their regulations had a major role to play as in defining the boundaries of sexual liberation for women. She says:

> In the nineteenth and early twentieth century, such sex-related institutions as family, motherhood, chastity, prostitution, birth control, and the double standard of morality had been subjected to feminist analysis by the "first wave" of feminists. Sexual repression had been privately acknowledged as a primary problem… "The first great work to be accomplished for woman is to revolutionize the dogma that sex is a crime.".… Though first-wave feminists did focus on the connection between the subjugation of women and male sexuality, for the most part they did not make women's sexuality central to their analysis of woman's social condition, except as it affected other institutions, like motherhood (Shulman 591).

In case of Uttara and Vasanti the problematic of motherhood are distinct on the ground of incapability to bear a child and longing and wish to grow a child as a motherly feeling. Vasanti began it as a revenge and lesson that she wanted to teach her sister but she was of course fond of Rajadhyaksha. The lack in case of Uttara becomes an experience of motherhood to Vasanti. It is the reason why she decides to bring up the child.

Vasanti never loved Rajadhyaksha and was preoccupied with the thought that she had to win over her sister; to devastate her. This characteristic of her nature was not limited to her sister only but extended to Rajadhyaksha too. She never told Rajadhyaksha that Dilip was his son. She thought that he would control her life as he would come to know about the child. She knew that he could never resist himself from reaching out his child. And once he manages to find access to his son, she feared that she would lose the control of her on her child. She felt the knowledge of truth becoming a trouble to her. She felt insulted when Rajadhyaksha came to Devdatt but never glanced at her. He would ignore her completely. Vasanti confesses that she wanted to be sure of her powers. She adds that once she became sure of them, she did not turn around to look at him.

The most peculiar feature of the desires of the characters in the play is vanity. The feelings understanding and realization of futility of all complex experience caused by certain behavioral traits of members of her family including herself, dawn on her. She advocates to putting an end to all the 'unceasing cycle of torment' and tells Vasanti to tell him about his son.

Rajadhyaksha dies before he listens to the news that he is the father of Dilip. This ultimately becomes a part of the sustenance of the vanity. It is not that they do not realize and understand the value of the thing they have lost. The lesson learned from it for lifetime however the lifetime is spent in the form of the upshot of the choice they made. Vasanti realizes her failure as soon she comes to know that Urmila has also abandoned Rajadhyaksha as she left the house.

The instigations to act against her own sister rose up to Vasanti as it was Uttara's ill treatment to her that caused various troubles about her very existence and self esteem. Vasanti says, "I didn't want to compete with you. But when you began to assume the pose of a patron, I decided … I'd defeat you … by taking away that one thing that gave you all your sense of power" (143).

Uttara's vanity is destroyed with knowledge that Dilip is Rajadhyaksha's son because Uttara maintains that she left him with all her dignity and honor unscathed. She believes that the world knows her as his wife and she never lost her prestige being so. She took everything that was rightfully hers.

It was only Rajadhyaksha who did not possess any grudge against none of the ladies. However both the women, in a way wished to cause pain to Rajadhyaksha. He replies to Vasudha the character in his novel, "I'm aware that I have wronged you. Charudutt gave you Pradeep. But in the novel, I made him my son whom Charudutt raised. But can I tell you the truth? I really wanted a son … I understand my mistake. I've changed a lot in thirty years" (149).

But it is Rajadhyaksha who felt hurt that Vasanti left him but he felt more hurt because she left him for someone whom he never appreciated on certain person grounds. Devdutt and Rajadhyaksha were in conflict on the issue like social responsibilities of an author. Pradnya asked him what he felt when Vasanti left him and went to live with Devdutt, Rajadhyaksha says, "I was unhappy. I felt insulted. She left me. I might have been able to digest that. But for whom? An ordinary, mediocre, unintelligent bohemian writer?" (135)

When Pradnya talks about breaking relationship with her boyfriend, Rajadhyaksha realizes what kind of mistake she is committing. He tells her not to break it since he experiences the result of breaking a relationship. He says that there is nothing as transient as human relationships. He tells her that the truth of a relationship should be confined to its moment. It doesn't cause pain then. He believes that we should be happy in receiving the amount of love though we get if for a moment.

The play *Autobiography* perhaps is the best attempt on the part of the writer to indicate the vanity of human wishes. It is not only in this play that Elkunchwar does attempt to present absurdity and meaninglessness of human relationship in all its complexities. It is always a moment that Elkunchwar seems to be presenting where human wishes contradict with what is being called as a common way of life. Sometimes it is confusion about valuing and giving importance to life or art or vice versa. This confusion leads Hemkant and Lalita's life to a destructive culmination. It indeed becomes a violent and horrible end for the couple and it gets too late for Hemkant to realize his mistake and make improvement upon it. Elkunchwar brings about the delicateness of such issues on a micro level. Rajadhyaksha's realization that his practice of writing literature, was never devoid of vanity and falsehood. It however dawned upon him as a result of lateral thinking. It could be called as the limitations of human experiences that the pressure of a situation allows very little time to contemplate about the action being taken by a human being regardless its profession or degree of maturity. It was Rajadhyaksha who wished Dilip could be his son as he loved to have a son but he could not have any and in the novel made Dilip his son. He admits that he wanted to have son and fulfills his desire so unknown to the fact that Dilip was his own son.

To write a novel about his life itself was an attempt to prove that he was right all the way in decisions he took. It was certainly the pressure he had to carry always of the grandeur of high human values that he vainly maintained in his life especially about nationalism and responsibilities of a writer. He received recognition and a prestigious place among the contemporary writers. The decision of writing the novel comes against this backdrop when the world knows his wife abandoned him and his wife's younger sister moves to stay with Devdutt. Rajadhyaksha could not bear the silence of a certain magnitude of meaning among his readers and society. In his novel thus Uttara and Vasanti become Urmila and Vasudha respectively. Devdutt becomes Charudutt. But he realizes the vanity of his desires and replies to Pradnya's question rather wisely about what he meant when he says he does not understand human relationships. She asks him whether he does not understand the relationships among the characters he develops in his writing or relationship in his real life. He replies, "Both. Or rather the relationships between my characters are the efforts I make to understand those that exist in my life" (133).

As he realizes the vanity of it more, he is afraid to talk as he fears whether he is capable of speaking truth. He says, "Why do we behave this way? Why do we live disguising lies as truth? I made Uttara's, Vasanti's, and my story so untrue! Conjuring up an imaginative truth to conceal my own lies. Or is there no truth in the world? Or does truth turn to lies when you don't understand it?" (150)

Uttara and Vasanti have deep instigations and motivations of their actions against Rajadhyaksha that are articulated actually at a fantasy level.

It is indeed a truth that Elkunchwar's *As One Discardeth the Old Clothes* … is the most subtle play that lays bare the reality of desire in its totality of life. There are six characters in the play Mukund, Sanjeevani and Bal are three children of Baba and Aai and there is a widow whom the family has given shelter after the death of her husband.

It exhibits whole problematic of the desire of a man that affects the whole family of his. It surpasses material objects of desires gradually as he approaches his death and waits for Raghu who could be a figure that he craved for his life. It is an abstract entity that every human being craves to achieve in the persuasion of happiness and completeness of his desires. It is the tireless chasing of one's life to find the completeness of meaning in one's life. In the case of Baba in the play, it has been Raghu who was the desired entity. But it remains however more abstract and unclear to himself as he could only describe him as a figure he could visualize when he was playing in mango grove, he fell from a tree and then saw Raghu for a moment. He searched then for him in the entire grove. But he disappeared. It happens twice in his life that he visualizes Raghu. Baba says, "Then again, once while swimming in the Morna, my feet suddenly cramped up and I was drowning unblinkingly from the shore. Somebody rescued me. After that I had sought him so often, foiling on the riverside. He was not to be found" (102-03).

Baba admits that it has been since his birth that his object of desire has been craving for a figure. He names it as Raghu that could be identified with the god Lord Krishna. It could have been the impact on his mind of the stories of Hindu gods and goddesses that could appear as forces that would seek to him ways of salvation. It is the hallucination that disturbed mind seeks under certain mental depression and problematic of mind. It is revealed to the audience only when Baba is on deathbed and his spiritual self can move freely on the stage while his body lays calm on the bed. He goes to everyone who talks but nobody can see or hear him.

It is with this technique Elkunchwar seeks the space where the character Baba reveals his desires that he otherwise could not have expressed. He reveals it on the two grounds that nobody is able to hear him and the second is that he realizes those are the last moments of his life and being his dear Raghu, the fear of hurting his loved ones is out of questions. It is here perhaps in the best manner the dramatist achieves the success of being able to reveal the mind of his character that speaks truth of his life. It is also unveiling the layers of positions taken by a human being as a member of society, family and position held in a structure influenced by social, political, economical and cultural factors.

He fell in love with Kaku in her marriage when he was already married. It had been only few days after his marriage the event happened and he decided that he would have her by any means. Madhu the husband of Kaku died on the second day of her marriage. Baba brought her home and provided her shelter. She too was in love with him since the time she eyed him in the marriage ceremony. He brought her home and always pined for her but never expressed his feelings of love to her for whole of his life. The desire was never expressed by either side. He also thought he brought her there needlessly. If he hadn't brought her here, she would have found a man for her somewhere else. But it is kept unspoken. Though he never confessed it to her, she could sense it and that was enough for her to fill her heart.

Baba's longing for her left her bigger void in the relationship between him and his wife. He could not associate himself with his wife completely. In the first place it was Raghu, his hallucination that busied his mind entirely and later on it was Kaku to whom his desires were engaged. This condition resulted in making Aai feel the loss of love she always felt. She always felt a detachment from him. She says coming closer to his body:

> My life was spent in yearning for you. My ears kept thirsting for just one call from you. But no. even at the most intimate moments my name never merged from your lips…Nothing moves me anymore. It is too late… You never asked for anything rightfully or demanded anything. Why didn't you ever show some possessiveness? Why did you never quarrel with

me? Why was this cold distance permanently between us? (109).

Human relations thus could never be a matter of study in isolation as it is a vivid reality that existence of single unit of problematic in certain individual results into creating disturbance in whole network of relationship that exists in relation with it. The lack of clarity adds the aura of mysticism, ignorance, meaninglessness, absurdity, unfulfilled lifelong longing for answer to questions in the mind. The life of an individual falls short of time to measure and recognize the change within the span of life time. It witnesses the changes of stages like teenage, youth, middle age and old age with addition to the responsibilities that keep on changing with time. It is with this impact Aai asks Baba:

> Or is there somebody else in mind?... Initially there was physical gratification. I agree. But my mind was never satiated. It always remained empty, starving. Neither my mind nor my body came to be fulfilled. Everything was mechanical, cold. Our children were born without love. When once I angrily asked you to stop all this, you stopped forever without any fuss. Didn't you really want to ever reach my mind? Whom did you have in mind? (109)

Aai always feared that he has Kaku in his mind. Due to this fear, she never left him alone in house. She always kept eye on her so that they do not get time in her absence to get attracted to each other. She never went to her parents fearing the consequences. But she never found a single moment when he did have inclinations towards Kaku nor it was found in Kaku's behavior. However it was systematically maintained by Baba that the care of children would be taken by Kaku as he insisted it was right as she was lonely woman and she needed the company of children but he admits that the real reasons were quite different. He confesses, "I abused your body a great deal. But there was always somebody else in mind" (96).

The feelings of lack of love in the mind of Aai drove her to seek the love somewhere out of the house and she did seek for that once vainly. It is in the relation, Sanju was begotten. She confesses that she could not find the solace there either and carried the weight whole of her life of the guilt and now that she wanted to confess to him that Sanjeevani is not his child. It was Sanjeevani he loved so deeply. He did everything he could do for her.

On other hand, he had a doubt that Bal is not his son. He could not ask her as the feelings of doubt would fill him with the feelings of guilt. He felt so ashamed of himself. Once he beat him for going for swimming but suddenly felt how he could get the right to beat him when he is not his blood. He really wanted to love him but he could really not love him due to the feelings that he is not his child. This detachment of him from his son Bal brought all negative feelings to him and he pines that he "[A]lways kept me at a distance. Never picked me up on your won. I would insist on coming close and sticking to you, and only then would you lift me onto your lap. But even then I could sense that your touch was cold" (104).

Bal always craved to be like his father. He grew with all his admiration for his father and the lack that he could not inherit anything of his father physically and psychologically. The level of influence had been so deep that he compared his married life with his parents and wished he could have such life.

In this way, the play *As One Discardeths the Old Clothes...* presents the possibility of complexity of human emotions and relations. What it adds to the knowledge of readers is, the understanding that creation of desire for someone could be a matter of utter uncertainty and devoid of logic. One could hardly make out the complete functioning of the origin of desire of one's own leave alone someone else's. It becomes clear that the desired end of a sexual desire does not always culminate into sexual union of two persons. Sex is not the act that in general sense is taken and considered as an end in itself. Though in modern times, considering sexual pleasure is taken an end itself and it has come to the terms of challenging the traditional point of views that sex is negative has to be avoided for free expression. It has not been a complete thesis. The longings of Baba on the death bed cross the boundaries, around which the complexity and lack of clarity of his desires existed. He craved for the widow for lifetime but never dared to express his desires.

The locus of human desire at times becomes a more difficult thing to trace. It is not the only matter that one cannot so easily find out and identify the origins of desires of a person as one does not always possess sufficient knowledge of human being as a psychoanalyst might demand information about the persons' childhood memories, dreams, habits, interests and so on. A piece of writing like that of a play does not always have a space to be occupied with necessary information. This 'lack' is a one side of the problem. The difficulty becomes graver with the understanding that a person most of the time does not understand motives of his or her own desires. It falls beyond his area of cognition to recognize in the first place how his desires for specific object, person or thing, are generated. Certain desires however could be recognized very easily as the result of certain circumstances, basic needs and those that often become the matter of familiarity in the course of time of life, whose existence could be recognized as natural and it anticipated. In the case of sexual desire however the nature of the matter becomes rather uncertain.

It has been always an important issue for the critics of literature and anthropologists like Levi Strauss who tried to present a poetics or a universal structure of incest relationships. Following its investigation, one reaches its various interpretations that hinges on specific factor like primitivism, culture, politics, social milieu, psychology, etc, or the practices indicating the amalgam of the all the factors mentioned above are also visible.

Observation regarding the role of fantasy in human psyche directing desires, behavior and activities with reference to Elkunchwar's *Desire in the Rocks* becomes a fruitful practice to understand the nature of desire. It is in connection with the incest relation between Lalita and Hemkant, the torture Lalita causes herself and the suicidal end Lalita instigates to herself and Hemkant. Fantasy could never receive a significant place among the frequently talked issues like conscious, unconscious, Oedipus complex, imagination, dreaming, psychosis, neurosis, wish fulfillment, etc. For Freud there exist conscious and unconscious fantasies. Let's bring a proper introduction to this issue.

Fantasies are a very essential part of our cognitive world. Fantasy, dreams are the components of our inner world. As long as they are in harmony with the outer world, we are lucky but a minor problem or inconvenience with them can bring us horrifying experience of nightmare and problematic world of experience.

Especially in the Age of Enlightenment, the role of fantasy in any creation was derogated. The poets like Coleridge declared a distinction between imagination and fantasy. For him fantasy was inferior to imagination. Fantasy was always denied of any role in creativity and was thought to be harmful to the capacity of human being for being able to produce serious and imaginative work of art and achieve uniformity of human psyche and world. It could also be traced back in ancient Greek when Plato used the term to mean it as a 'purely mental activity that did not have relationship with external reality'. After him Aristotle used the term with slightly different meaning and it was used with the little difference from time to time. However, its disconnection from reality or rational view of reality was maintained. The view never allowed fantasy to perceive any serious attention. The result was that the creative side of fantasy was never given importance.

Freud used the term in psychoanalyses and the original German term used by him was "die Phanasie", and the related verb was "phantasieren". He used the words to denote conscious fantasies and pre-conscious fantasie- the once conscious and then changed into unconscious "phantasies" – and to phantasies which, according to him have always been unconscious. In the course of time it has created many problems. Antony Easthope in his book *The Unconscious* says, "For psychoanalysis fantasy means: 1) an imaginary scene or narrative; 2) in which the person fantasizing is present: 3) but a scene altered or disguised; 4) so as to fulfill a wish" (Easthope 110).

Lalita comes to the terms of killing herself. It happens only when she realizes that her brother does not love her and he has messed it with his concept of art. It is why her mind is full of thoughts of guilt, loss, the curse of the beggar, self destruction as to get the punishment for the sin she has committed. The existence of complex and phobic situations in which Lalita lives since her childhood, have prompted her to think it.

> Lalita: You're older than me. By fifteen years. That's why I feel scared. I've spent all these twenty years of my life just being scared.
>
> Hemkant: Were you afraid of Dadasaheb.
>
> Lalita: Petrified. After he died, I thought I was free of fear. But then the trustees and solicitors came. I was afraid of them. I couldn't understand what they were

saying. Then you came, Hem. And I felt really free (Elkunchwar 72).

It had been quite late for Lalita to come to the realization of the freedom she anticipated. The fears and suppression she lived with since her childhood had affected her mind too deeply. What made her continue her life living and wait for her messiah to come, were her fantasies. It included both the conscious and unconscious. The problem with them got her into the destructive end. It could be said so because fantasy realizes a desire in a systematic way or

> "rather, its function is similar to that of Kantian 'transcendental schematism': a fantasy constitutes our desire, provides its co-ordinates; that is, it literally 'teaches us how to desire'… fantasy meditates between the formal symbolic structure and the positivity of the objects we encounter in reality – that is to say, it provides a 'schema' according to which certain positive objects in reality can function as objects of desire, filling in the empty places opened up by the formal symbolic structure" (Zizek 7).

The entry of the brother and sister into the *wada* brings the feeling of fear to Lalita and she could easily connect it with the dark time she lived in. The feelings of guilt, sin, betrayal, renunciation that led the tragic end of the duo had been the outcome of the disturbance of the 'schema' Lalita maintained. It included her brother as lover as it is how her world of fantasy realized a desire and solace and in a way it was at the same time an escape into and results of the dreadful childhood memories. This could be the answer to the question of incest. Hemkant as the result of the prevailing conditions functioned as an object of desire. The aftermath of it, relates oneself (Lalita) in contrast with religion, God, social norms that could also bring about violent responses to one self and to others as well. So it means in a way, fantasy not only tells how to desire but also appropriate other feelings once the specific object is desired. Thus result could be in renunciation of one's own child or body:

> Lalita: It's like a patch of leukoderma that has spread over the whole body. A few days of shame, but when the whole body is covered, what shame can there be? Sin once. Then it's over. That's not how it is. Sin never ends (Elkunchwar 115).

The consequences of incest relationship in almost all cultures are negative. The main reason behind it is the way the codes of conduct in the human relationships are structured and evolved through times. After the evidence of destructive end of Hemkant and Lalita in the mansion, we realize that the culmination that occurs as the result of such relation is due to not only that it comes against the socially accepted ways of behavior and conduct and society punishes such intrusion, unfamiliar and unaccepted gesture, but also it has the share of personal histories, psychologies and concept of love. The actual conflict in life commences when the maintained gestures are broken or shaken. Human beings tend to maintain a structure of ideas that takes for granted many things, results, culminations that they anticipate and the stronger the structure of such ideas, longer they hold on the views and lead a life in the same direction. It is only with the conflict with the maintained structure of ideas, the minds of human beings are fractured and they are left with such state of mind when violence, death, depression, struggle, agitation, breaking of hearts and many other such negative results could be anticipated. However, it occurs only with the conflict with the structure. It does not always happen that the very base of it is shaken so easily. It requires an event that could be socially, economically, psychologically, politically or historically instigated. In the process an individual arrives at a realization that the anticipation and the very base of structure are not real or the other person or entity has disrespected it. At such times, the individual like Lalita, cannot always prepare themselves for an other way of life as an acceptance of such possibility. That such behavior could be expected in most of day to day life situations but in this case it does not appear that simple as the problematic after the realization fortifies since the structure of the ideas had already become the way of their life and the very part of their psyche that thinks and anticipates things in a specified way. The shakes to the view do not instantly offer them a way out. They undergo an experience of agony and trauma.

In his article entitled "The Indian Oedipus", A. K. Ramanujan declares that it is so easy to find a parallel example where a son marries his mother and kills his father. He tells that the Indian writers while defining the incestuous sin of intercourse with a *guru's* wife, they add a list of other sins 'of the same form' or 'equal'. He quotes Nicholas (1976: 16) who emphasizes from the *Naradasmriti.*

> If a man has sexual intercourse with any of these women viz. mother, mother sister, mother-in-law, a wife of a paternal uncle or a friend or a pupil, a sister, a sister's friend, daughter-in-law, the wife of one's Vedic teacher, a woman of the same gotra (clan), one who has come for protection, a queen, an ascetic woman, one's wet-nurse, a woman performing a *vrata* (vow) and a *brahmana* woman, he becomes guilty of the sin of the violator of the guru's bed (i.e., incest). For that crime no other punishment is laid down except that of cutting the penis (Quoted in Ramanujan 121).

In the play *Flower of Blood,* there are four characters and it opens at such time when the couple Bhau and Padma who have lost their young son and have a young daughter Leelu who studies at school. Raja is a paying guest at their house who is a student studying in a college. The complexity of the relationship among these characters grows more complex with the confusion of the mother's longing for her lost son and finding a solace of the love in Raja and for Bhau it had been the loss of the son and wife's and daughter's inclination towards Raja puts him in psychological trouble and the love of Leelu for Raja makes it more complex.

The Oedipal Complex takes more influential form than that of love and Bhau's regime as a father. Maternal ego and daughter's love feeling for Raja encounters and they being the most antagonist about each other cannot thus resolve into positivity of culmination. It seeks its origin in already established formal symbolic structure of relationships. The complexity and unacceptability of the relationships including that of incest emerge due to the way human psyche realizes the desire and fulfills it and it tends to function in such a manner where it does not follow the regulations set by the certain culture and its ideology. The social order is governed by the set of ideas in a certain period of time and its ideological forces have strong disciplinary ideas of control especially about sexuality. It does not allow any challenge to its formal symbolic order. This established order is enacted from the certain positions like religious, political and economic nature. While the realization of a desire by an individual is governed by "a 'schema' according to which certain positive objects in reality can function as objects of desire, filling in the empty places opened up by the formal symbolic structure" (Zizek 7).

This idea has been taken help of while analyzing the nature of the incest relationship between Lalita and Hemkant in the play *Desire in the Rocks.* It had been the case of incest

relationship between the brother and the sister. In the play
Flower of Blood the object of desire is appropriated in certain
form. The maternal love for son comes naturally under the
same category but in the play the loss of the son is attempted
to recover by offering the affection to male child and he does
not happen to be a child from any close relationship. The
substitution found by the maternal ego in the form of Raja
could be called as a peculiar characteristic of human psyche
especially that of female one. The substitution for the desired
object of desire is sought in different forms in order to receive
the same happiness and pleasure out of it. It works on both
levels of wisdom and unconscious.

In case of the love of Padma for Raja it works on the both
levels and is predominantly governed by the feeling of loss of
her original son. The realization of the loss becomes frequent
point of discomfort in the process of longing for the love from
Raja as a son. It clearly suggests the extreme possibility of
appropriation of the object of desire in reality. And Raja the
object in reality like any other human being find it strange
why Padma does not charge him for staying there as a paying
guest and why she tidies up his room. Padma however does not
give to the imbalances like that of illogic and lack of reasoning.
She tells Raja, "Dear, dear Raja, you will never understand
this deep, deep affection that we women feel. If your mother
comes here some day, I'll tell her, give me your son, I'd like to
adopt him" (Elkunchwar 38). Besides the many things that
bring complexity to the desire of the mother for the boy Raja,
Padma's understanding of Raja as a child of someone else is
clear. Her desire is full of reason and makes the strategies to
treat him as her own son and at the same time to take care
that he does not get fed up with it. She tells Raja to stay in the
house and never to leave it. According to her we need people
to fill our house. When she tells Raja about her son Shashi and
how he wanted to have a big house. She mentions that Shashi

"alone would have filled it, with his vitality, with his presence" (Elkunchwar 39). This emotional account of her becomes one of the strategies of her. It is both planned and result of certain unconscious traits of her mind caught in the frustration of the loss and it attempts to acquire a substitute pleasure for it.

This leads to a condition where Leelu does not respond to her mother very well for the both reasons that her mother always scolds her for small things and spends more time with Raja and on the other hand she causes troubles to Bhau also. The one of the major reasons of the complexity mentioned above could be traced to her realization that it is time for her menopause. The realization of it troubles the mind of Padma. It is commonly seen in women in their forties and fifties. Whenever it gets late for her periods, her mood sways. The realization of this possibility brings with it the loss of hope and capability to become a mother again for Padma. It is something that a woman amidst the regime of various forces and responsibilities takes pride in possessing. It is the capacity to be able to create and becoming the source of the creation. It is not so easy for Padma to handle the pressure of the various forces while her mind is already tormented by the loss of her son. When she wishes to fulfill her desire for a child and also to seek a lover in the son who is not of hers, the understanding of the reality however does not leave her at ease. Though she tries to hold on the boy, it becomes irritating for the boy to cope up with it. The swaying of her mood is fanatic and irresistible due to the fact of the loss. It does not however again mean that she would have behaved in the same manner if her son were alive. It was she who let Shashi to join the army. Padma admits to Raja, "But I don't understand myself. Am I wrong or are the others wrong? How should I behave? I don't seem to find anything interesting. Nothing attracts me. I keep wondering what I am doing, and for what or for whom" (Elkunchwar 54). The next thing she does is another attempt of regaining and asserting a moment of pleasure when she complains to Bhau that he has a wife and she has desires and expectations.

It becomes more complex for Padma to manage the pressure and it results into psychological abnormality like that of writing sort of love letter addressed to nobody but relive the experience of love that once she lived happily. The reluctant desire of Bhau in their early period of marriage also plays negative role in the construction of her psyche. It leaves her in a certain state of mentality where she craves for the pleasure. It will not be more suitable to say the loss of an only son was the only cause that was responsible for Padma's disturbed behavior. It is connected to various relationships she has in the family besides the memories of her son, her marriage, her youth, the signs of old age, etc. She cannot tolerate the idea of Leelu talking to Raja and suddenly takes the decision to tell Raja to find another room for him. The way the possibility of adopting Raja as her son is broken down with the realization of his mother being alive and loving him intensely; it is with the same sudden internal compulsion she abandons the idea of possibility of new child immediately after she expresses her desire to Bhau. Bhau asks her whether she wants divorce from him so that at least then she can live happily. But Leelu finds out the letters in her room and calls her mother "a dirty woman". It comes as an embarrassing situation for Padma. It becomes almost impossible for her to make Bhau think the condition in which such fake love letters were written. And finding it impossible to explain she breaks down saying:

> Don't be angry, please. These letters, they're not even real letters. Look. Take a look at them. All of them. Look, they are not even addressed to anybody. They weren't written with anybody in mind. They were just something to do. Something to keep me busy. I used to get so bored… I'm not what you think I am. I am

really not. I'm really not like that. Forgive me, please.
I have no one. Please don't leave me (Elkunchwar 60).

Desire, saying it in a more generalized way, forms a base for
almost every kind of problem and complexity of relationship;
it is the desire which becomes the source of solution to the
problem. In the first place, it is the cause of problem and in the
second it is the panacea. The loss of desire ultimately results in
ultimate destruction. It is the destruction at the core. A person
like Padma engulfed in psychological complexities finds it very
difficult to come out of it and live life normally. It is the people
around her who can offer real comfort and realization of her
troubles and her vain attempts get involved in certain bondages
due to their personal lives and engagements. It happens with
many people suffering from psychological disorders. Padma
attempts to tighten her grip on the situation to control it but
it tends to slip away with her strength. The too much affection
irritates Raja; Leelu is tired of her lectures and scolding and
husband feels more pity for her and loses desire for her. The
reactions that Leelu and Bhau give when Padma appears in
front of them in the sari, make her feel that she has done
something abnormal that she is not supposed to do.

There are two things that happen in process of realizing
a desire by a tormented person like Padma. First the person
tends to seek immediate happiness out of the direct way
of receiving pleasure. It could be for Padma by cleaning
the room of Raja or just lying down on his bed keeping
the lights off. Though it is momentarily, such ways are
sought in order to get rid of the pressure building up in one's
mind. There remains a very little time to think logically
and plan systematically before one acts to avoid the growing
complexity of web of thinking about certain matter at hand.
Secondly, it is the burden of realization that people around
one, have noticed one doing the crazy thing. In case of

Padma, it is wearing the sari or writing the letter leaves her beyond explanation. This remains in mind and brings about feeling of guilt making the person feel more depressed. But what keep this complex play goes on moving is desire of human beings for something. The time when such desires die out completely, the human psychology becomes impossible to find comforts in normality of the world. Unlike Padma, Lalita finds her resolution of the complexity grown in her mind in suicide in *Desire in the Rocks*.

Elkunchwar's *Holi* describes the conflict of the students studying in a college and staying at hostels at college campus. Elkunchwar's this play becomes perhaps the first play that points the situation of the growing intolerance among the youngster studying at college and registering their protest against the institutionalization and authoritative regimes hailing from different systems. The homosexual desire between Shrivastav and Anand marks the visibility of gay relationship between the two distinctively. At times it seems to be at the core of the thematic concern of the play since it is the concerns that instigate the major course of action in the play. It is out of this desire Anand reports the name of the students creating mess in the program organized by the principal on the day of *Holi*. It ultimately results in torture to Anand by the group of students and suicide of Anand.

Hoshang Merchant in introduction to the book *Yarana: Gay Writing from India* writes about the development of the study in concern with homosexuality and how it exited from the time unknown but silence was always maintained on the issue like incest and other taboo relationships. He says that there is no such beast in zoology as a 'homosexual'. He talks about the etymology of the word and says that it is an invention of late nineteenth century European science, half Greek (Grk. 'homo' = 'same') and half Latin ('sexual' being Latin in root). He explains that

It denotes not a person but a category that several sensitive persons, obliging science, have tried to fit themselves into. NRI gays in *Trikone* (San Jose, California) have concocted a terminology for Gays: 'Samlingan' for the sexuality, 'samlingia' for 'homosexual', i.e., a literal translation of Western terms. Such a term does not exist in India where the practice is not codified, only quietly condoned and above all, not talked about. As Foucault reminds us in *History of Sexuality,* sex is not modern, talking about it is (Marchant xi).

Having thus realized a state of study regarding the homosexuality in Indian context from the expert of the book by Marchant that offers the true account of homosexual experience by the people in India, it helps us in investigating the relationship between Shrivastav and Anand who share a room in the hostel. Elkunchwar describes the relationship with certain passing references that occur in the conflict the students have with college authority. Anand loves Shrivastav and is more involved with him than Shrivastav. The way he treats Anand suggests that he has his interests of different kinds. For Shrivastav he is the source to gain monetary and other benefits out the emotional attachment. He at times threatens him if Anand does not get ready to offer him the things he demands from him. When Anand complains to him about why he sold his sunglasses, Shrivastav tell him that he is going to change the room. Anand cannot bear the thought of Shrivastav changing his room. He replies, "I'll kill myself!" (Elkunchwar 10) Shrivastav deploys this strategy in order to get five rupees from him.

What however matters in this regard is not how the both develop the homosexual relationship. It is of more concern that the homosexual desire does exist and the play has its visibility. Anand faces more troublesome remarks from other student friends of him for his intimacy with Shrivastav. It does not detain him from keeping its exhibition of concern for Shrivastav limited to himself. It is more interesting to find out the strangeness of the relationship when one partner does not respond to the other respectively and it is known to the person loving the other. Though the text does not offer detailed discourse on the construction of homosexual identity of Anand, it remains to see the factors that promote him to assert his homosexual desire for Shrivastav. He goes at the extent that in order to save him from the strict disciplinary actions, he goes to the principal and reports the names of the students involving the trouble at the program and deliberately excludes the name of Shrivastav.

Hoshang Merchant in his quote as mentioned above makes the mention of Foucault and it poses a question regarding the suitability and authenticity of application of the western theories to sexuality in Indian context. In this regard Janaki Nair and Mary John write:

> We cannot, but draw upon western theories, since they determine at an unconscious level, the reading practices we bring to bear on our work. But this till leaves us with the task of theories action, which can never take the form of the application of a theory that one possesses in advance, but must resemble a process, a historical and political mode of conceptualizing sexual economics that would be true to our experience of an uneven modernity, calling for multiple levels of analysis and the forgiving of articulation between the global and the local (Quoted in Narrain and Bhan 7).

The homosexual desire in the play could thus be analyzed with the help of the basic framework of western theories like that of Foucault bringing down the forces like patriarchy, power, knowledge, reason and religion. What makes the personal and contextual experience of the analyses altogether a different practice of realization of new notions that go into making the reality of experience of homosexuality in Indian context is the very framework of history, tradition, memory, culture and social norms that underlie the life style of the people at a certain period of time. It involves the conscious acknowledgment to the issues like psychology, politics, economics, history, sociology and the process of cultural identification. And they are time specific and cannot always be isolated from its local and national relevance and significations.

One of the reasons that could be cited regarding the reluctance of Shrivastav in the homosexual desire other than his disinterestedness is the way in which the common thought is prevalent about the sexuality. It is labeled as dirty and outrageous. Foucault in *The History of Sexuality Vol.I* puts it in the following way:

> As defined by the ancient civil or canonical code, sodomy was a category of forbidden acts; their perpetrator was nothing more than the juridical subject of them. The nineteenth century homosexual becomes a personage, a past, a case history and childhood, in addition to bring a type of life, a life form, and morphology, with an indiscreet anatomy and possibly a mysterious physiology (Foucault 43).

The mention of such sexuality in Vatsyayana's *Kamsutra* and other canonical texts produced on the subject shows the existence of such practices. The texts never does approve of the relationships. It however does not become only the subject to the disapproval by the common subject but it becomes the part of regulatory body that legalizes the rules of code of conduct in a certain matter of relationship. It is here identification of the areas is done and as a necessity they are defined in a very clear way and it tends to culminate into certain practices of overlooking, undermining, ignoring, generalization, politics, cultural and religious dogmatism, etc. The section 377 of *Indian Penal Code* drafted in 1860 by Lord Macaulay contains:

> Whoever voluntarily has carnal intercourse against the order of nature with any man, woman or animal shall be punished with imprisonment... which may extend to 10 years and shall be liable to fine. Explanation: Penetration is sufficient to constitute the carnal inter course necessary to the offence described in this section (Narrain and Bhan 7).

As mentioned above here is an example how the generalization in a legal way of defining misses certain possibilities of more forms of 'queer' relationships. It calls such desire as "sexual acts against the order of nature". In Indian context the law clearly states the nature of crime of sexual kind. It talks about the sexual acts against the order of nature. It is homosexual acts even of it is consensual and in private. It is the reason Ashwini Sukthankar, in her introduction to *Facing the Mirror: Lesbian writing in India* (1999) points out the exemption of lesbians in Indian law. She knows that it is not out of any kind of privilege but out of contempt and ignorance. She is not happy about the nonexistent nature of Indian lesbianism. She writes:

> ...we don't live outside the law, as gay men do in our country, we live between the lines. 'Section 377' of the Indian Penal code makes homosexual acts between men illegal but it does not have technically have lesbianism in its purview, since he legal definition of intercourse requires penetration (Sukthankar xiv).

It is the death of Anand that puts the end to his life so condemned by his fellow companions. The inclinations he has towards Shrivastav could never be understood by the students other than a way that could not be called as normal and accepted. No one seems to acknowledge the possibility of homosexual relationship. Nevertheless it is also to be taken into account the positivity of development of consciousness regarding the matter in the form of writing by a writer like Elkunchwar.

Works Cited

Adiga, Arvind. *The White Tiger*. New Delhi: Harper Collins, 2008. Print.

Chakroborty, Kaustav, ed. *Indian Drama in English*. New Delhi: PHI Learning Pvt. Ltd., 2011. Print.

Dattani, Mahesh. *Collected Plays. Vol. II*. New Delhi: Penguin Books India, 2005. Print.

"Desire." Def. 2b. *Oxford Advanced Learner's Dictionary*. 8th ed. 2010. Print.

Easthope, Antony. *The Unconscious*. Oxon: Routledge, 2009. Print.

Elkunchwar, Mahesh. *Collected Plays of Mahesh Elkunchwar Vol. I*. New Delhi: Oxford University Press, 2009. Print.

Elkunchwar, Mahesh. *Collected Plays of Mahesh Elkunchwar Vol. II*. New Delhi: Oxford University Press, 2011. Print.

Foucault, Michael. *The History of Sexuality. Vol. I*. New York: Vintage Books. 1990. Print.

Hall, Kristy. *The Stuff of Fantasy*. London: Karnac Books Ltd. 2007. Print.

Merchant. Hoshang. *Yarana: Gay Writings from India*. New Delhi: Penguin, 1999. Print.

Narrain, Arvind. *Queer'despised Sexuality: Law and Social Change*. Bangalore: Books for Change Pub. 2004. Print.

Narrain, Avind, and Gautham Bhan. ed. *Because I Have a Voice: Queer Politics in India*. New Delhi: Yodha Press. 2005. Print.

Jahagirdar, Chandrashekhar. "Marathi Drama After 1960." *Haritham* 5 (1995):64. Print.

Machiavelli. *The Prince*. Trans. C. E. Detmold. Kent:1997. Print.

Rakesh, Mohan. *Halfway House*. New Delhi: OUP. 1990. Print.

Shinde, Tarabai. *Stri-Purush Tulana*. Ed. Nagnath Kottapalle. Aurangabad: Kailash Publication. 2010. Print.

Ramanujan, A. K. "The Indian Oedipus." *Vishnu on Freud's Desk: A Reader in Psychoanalysis and Hinduism*. ed.T.G. Vaidyanathan and Jeffery J. Kripal, New Delhi:Oxford University Press. 1999. Print.

Salunkhe. A.H. *Astikshiromani: Charvak*. Satara: Lokayat Prakashan, 1992. Print.

Scruton, Roger. *Sexual Desire*. New York: Continuum, 2006. Print.

Shirly, Sidney. "Sexuality Versus Psychology: A Study of Mahesh Elkunchwar's *Garbo* and *Desire in the Rocks*". *Journal of English Language and Literature 2:1*(2015): 124. Web. 12 Oct, 2015. Print.

Shulman, Alix Kats. "Sex and Power: Sexual Bases of Radical Feminism." *Signs* 5:4 (1980): 591. JSTOR. Web. June, 2011.

Sukthankar, Ashwini. *Facing the Mirror: Lesbian Writings from India*. New Delhi: Penguin, 1999. Print.

Vatsyayana. *Kamasutra*. Trans. Richard Francis Burton. New Delhi: Penguin Evergreens, 1862. Print.

Zizek, Slovej. *Pervert's Guide to Cinema*. www.youtube.com, youtube, mp4, *2005*. Web. 20 May, 2010.

…,. *The Plague of Fantsies*. London: Verso, 1997. Print.

Chapter III
'REVOLT' IN THE SELECT PLAYS OF MAHESH ELKUNCHWAR

Liberty, that nightingale with the voice of a giant, muses the most profound sleepers. . . How is it possible to think of anything today except to fight for or against freedom? Those who cannot love humanity can still be great as tyrants. But how can one be indifferent?

Ludwig Boerne, February 14, 1983

Literature has been an important tool to register various responses of mankind and the stimulus for all kinds of the responses has been of different nature and origins. Unfortunately history of civilization has been the history of subjugation, injustice and imperialism. These vital issues have the characteristics of economic and political nature and they somehow still form the core of human affairs. Literature, in a way, is an expression not only with the view and intention of writing of course of incidents and events in a certain literary form but it is the inevitability of the expression as a result of the conflict of two or many entities. It would be not difficult to see how there has been inevitability of the conflict since the time unknown. The dialectics could never be an ineffective characteristic of the changes that have marked the beginning and end of various phenomena.

There is a glorious tradition of the literature that could be called as the literature of conflict or literature of revolt. The revolt could be defined as the instant reaction to the certain change, action, process or behavior. Agitation, defense, protection, violence are some of the features of revolt. The first decade of twentieth century also witnessed the strong undercurrent of the literature of revolt beginning with the literature of revolutionary ideas of nationalism to the *Dalit* Literature of revolt against the atrocities against *dalits* in India. *Dalit* literature and tribal literature marked the major development in last decades of twentieth century in Marathi literature. It also marked the beginning of a luminous literature of revolt in entire India. It presented altogether new aesthetics of its own. Its impact had been remarkable and it governed the literary scene of Indian literature for more than three decades and caused much discussion on various levels. Though it had its origin in political and social movements, *Dalit* autobiographies, memoirs, testimonies, etc became an effective tool of the writers to express their experience and saga of pain through the type of narration. One of the reasons of the great authenticity of the literature was involved in the fact that the people writing the testimonies or autobiographies were not writers by profession but the ordinary common people who happened to express their experiences in life through the medium of written form.

Feministic literature, colonial and post colonial literature, African colonial and post colonial literature, socialist or Marxist literature are in a strongest sense of meaning the literature of revolt. It has been the revolt of different nature. The causes of the revolt are different and have received the stimuli from various sources but the common feature of the revolt is that it acts against the subjugation that the 'other' had to suffer from for ages. The layers of the suppression are of myriad folds. Women and *dalit* were doubly suppressed whereas the *dalit* women were triply suppressed due to the multiple nature of suppression embedded in the form of gender, caste, religion and patriarchal discrimination. It is interesting to observe that *dalit* literature was effective in certain forms like poetry and autobiographies only. Feminism and post colonial literature were in vogue mainly through the fictional writings that flourished in the second part of twentieth century.

It is true that we are able to concentrate on certain strong epoch making types of literary presentations. Such presentations vary time to time. The way the subject matter of the expression and presentation matter, the observation also reveals how there had been a specific choice of certain genre among fiction, poetry and drama. However such strong undercurrent at least for short period of time blinds us to the other forms of streams of human expression. There are many factors of course that decide on the popularity and the flux of development of the form of writing through discussion and expression through critical and creative format. As a part of amalgam of whole literature produced in a specific time, every trend, that human experience registers, matters in order to arrive at the understanding of human nature and culture.

Drama is one of the most significant and effective form of writings that has proved many times fruitful in expressing and achieving its impact on society. It has been effective in conveying the message it wants due to the nature of the presentation in dialogic form and more importantly the facility and advantage of dramatic presentation on the stage.

It is evident how religion has made use of this form of expression from the beginning in the types like morality and miracle play and in Indian context it was presentations like *Nautanki* which had majority of themes of expression from religious text like the *Mahabharat* and the *Ramayan*. In the recent times, theatre has been viewed as the place for more opportunities to achieve the desired ends of the intention of the writing. Brecht looked on theatre as a means of social change. The socialist and Marxist perspectives always attempted to make theatre as a place of experiments so that more effective form of expression could be found out in order to quicken the process of the desired change.

When talked about the revolt in the dramatic writings of Elkunchwar, they exhibit such tendencies of two kinds. One is that of the selection of subject matter for his writing which predominantly characterizes the expression of feelings that have been tabooed and prohibited. Secondly his writings in their totality are a form of revolt as compared against the backdrop of the Marathi dramatic writings before 1960s.

Since 1960s the change that took over the various forms of Marathi had been more prominent. Dramatic writings changed radically since then. It changed on two levels; one is that the plays started to be written with great precision and professional theatres were strengthened and secondly the playwrights began to handle subjects of innovative nature that eventually enriched whole tradition of dramatic writing in the language. The newness of the change lied in the detachment of them from the tradition of conservative writing that never attempted the thematic concern that would connect to the larger implications of literature on the universal level.

Dr. Supriya Pendhari observes in her book *Marathi Natyasrushtitil Vidroh ani Navata* that in world of Marathi theatrical writing Khanolkar, Tendulkar and Elkunchwar are some of those playwrights who represented the Marathi theatrical writing scenes more vitally than others could do in the thematic concerns and subjects.

Revolt in the present connection however is conceived and realized on two important levels. One as an act of a playwright that becomes in intself an act of revolt due to its newness; its ability to break down the established social, political and creative norms; it is the revolt that has entire ability to bring about a new tradition in the existing ways of doing literature. Tendulkar and Elkunchwar have ushered in an era in Marathi dramatic writing that marked the beginning of an age of revolution. The nature of this revolution however was not limited to the matter of opposing the old tradition or it was not the mere result of the thinking against the traditional conservatism and totalitarianism. Both the dramatists had in their background the reservoir of information and knowledge of European and American tradition of theatrical writings and trends among them. This fact could be supposed as the crucial feature. It brought later on to many new Marathi writers, the understanding of various advancement that took place in different parts of the world and contributed to the overall knowledge of human nature.

Tendulkar brought a shock to the minds of Marathi People with the characters like Sakharam from *Sakharam Binder*, Shivappa from *Baby* or Ghashiram from *Gharshiram Kotwal*, Leela Benare from *Silence! The Court is in Session*. These are however some of the selective examples of the personae that represent a social psyche. They come upon the scene to propagate not only its existence but also to reveal that it is a form in itself that has grown out of shape. It rather asserts its existence and possesses the ability to make a human mind give thoughts to it and the complexity of its existence. The contribution of Tendulkar to the Marathi theatre in particular and Indian theatre in general has been immense.

In Sri Ram Memorial Lectures, Tendulkar narrates his lifelong involvement in theatre as follows;

> What I like about those years is that they made me grow as a human being. And theatre which was my major concern has contributed to this in a big way. It helped to analyze life – my own and lives of others. It led me to make newer and newer discoveries in the vast realm of the human mind that still defies all available theories and logic... Now I am aware of what I am doing while I do it. I am my own audience and the critic, if one may use the language of the theatre (Chakroborty 118).

Elkunchwar in his *Yatanaghar* and *Desire in the Rocks* dealt with the subject of incest and it had been basically too daring way of selection of subject matter to such audience who could never imagine such thing to be written and would personally prefer silence on the subject. It has two aspects one that incest is still considered as a taboo and is less talked about. Silence is major practice observed whenever there is a scope of talk or discussion on it. It begins right from the informal situations in the family and perhaps it is the significant place that looks after the security of such silence is maintained.

Garbo is about a prostitute and three friends of her, who have physical relation with her and the complicated relation that results into the murder of Garbo the prostitute. In *Autobiography*, reality of human desire is revealed. In *Holi* resistance of a student community against the authority that denies them holiday, is registered. The form of their revolt has many characteristics like that of violence and destruction. Elkunchwar does not however miss to offer the account of the homosexual desire in the play. The visibility of it however is a pure form of revolt that has multi layers of resistance to the gendered self and voices against the authority that insists the conformity.

In the play *As One Discardeth Old Clothes...*, Elkunchwar presents to us the last moments of a person on deathbed who realizes the futility of man's existence and the form of revolt he adopts is becoming one with God and at the same time denying and breaking himself free from the relationship that he tried in vain throughout his life to bring a satisfactory meaning. In *Party* Elkunchwar reveals the psyche of middle class set of people who represent different profession in the society. He depicts the hypocrite nature of the people in their vanity of wishes and meaningless pursuit for popularity. The character of Amrit in the play represents the consciousness in the society that believes in working for social cause. He believes that the movement against social and political injustice could not be defeated unless one brings about the revolt in the active form. He believes that the passive forms like that of writing and philosophizing issues are mere vain attempt of dreaming of the change.

Mahesh Elkunchwar in his *Wada* trilogy i.e. *Old Stone Mansion, Pond* and *Apocalypse* brings out the strong image of the pond that defines the dissatisfaction of the major male characters like Chandu, Parag and Abhay. Elkunchwar here presents perhaps in the most effective form the existential struggle of human beings and their lifelong struggle to belong to certain space. The vanity of the life experiences and desires; their meaninglessness and inability of them being capable to offer solace to minds of individuals, eventually takes the shape of a revolt against them. It results into the systematic attempt of establishing oneself in either a nostalgic or an abstract or a material form of symbolism so that extremity of conflicts in the minds could be pacified. It automatically becomes an event that offers solution to the internal and external struggle of the mind and body. And most importantly it offers the space to human psyche to feel at ease at least for time being.

Handling of the themes like prostitution, sexuality, incest, homosexuality, activism, suicide, death, futility of Indian marriage system, disappointment of the youth against the political and rigid democratic systems and man's perpetual existential conflict with the notions of dissatisfaction, meaninglessness, longing to belong to a certain space, indicates the variety of issues with which Elkunchwar makes an impact on the Marathi theatre. These conflicts represent the typical forms of resistance and revolt. The subjects that receive the treatment in the plays of Elkunchwar however have the characteristics of novelty, different manner of presentation and the skillfulness of using the space of stage to present the subject matter considering its scope and limitations.

It will not be naïve generalization when it is summed up saying that the plays of Elkunchwar succeeds in making the audience and readers consider and ponder over the subject matter of his plays mainly due to the revolutionary nature of human affairs he depicts in the fabric of the story. Though violence, ideological conflicts, deterioration of the Indian family system, sexuality, psychological complications, loss of identity, longing for meaning of life, suicide and death have formed the basis of the main action of various plays of Elkunchwar, they have the existence of them without any sort of repetition and resemblance with other subject matter. The revolt and the conflict with the themes have been presented by the dramatist with no artificial assertion or longing for certain impact on audience. Of course *Garbo* is an exception to it. It happens in the case of Elkunchwar due to the notion of inspiration for writing a play. He does not believe in numbers.

Speaking on the necessity of revolt and conflict as an answer to the charges of pessimism on him, Tendulkar says "[m]y experience of my times, my life, has shown me that the individual is largely disempowered, made abject, reduced to the groupings" (Chakroborty 117).

The identification of the inspirations and the stimuli of a writer behind writing a piece of literary work is not an easy job for any critic. Problematic of this notion begins right from the authority of the author in claiming the importance of becoming the core in the process of creation and holding the capability and ability to control the work of art and modulate its impact as a result of his/her individual efforts. However it is not always impossible to make out the nature of the time in which the work of art is written and also to identify the possibility of the existing elements that are likely to participate in the process of stimulation. The description of the process becomes difficult due to basic complex nature of the phenomena ruling the contemporary time. The responsible elements and ingredients for forming stimuli to regulate the process of writing get intermingled and grow more complicated due their inseparable nature assimilation with other elements. In his book *The Age of Revolution 1789 - 1848* Eric Hobsbawm observes such type of assimilation and calls it 'dual revolution' and says:

> If a single misleading sentence is to sum up the relations of artist and society in this era, we might say that the French Revolution inspired him by its example, the Industrial Revolution by its horror, and the bourgeois society, which emerged from both, transformed his very existence and modes of creation (Hobsbawm 255).

In *Holi* a group of students who stays at hostel, is unhappy because the principal of their college has not declared a holiday on the day of *Holi*. The presence of various issues that make the students revolt against the principal of the college, notifies the consciousness of the students. It represents almost omnipresent conditions at educational system in Maharashtra. As the play begins and the students come to know that the principal did not declare a holiday and besides it he has organized a talk by speaker who is an 'authority' on the subject of Hindu religion and Indian culture, the language used by the students from the beginning of the play suggests the powerful hatred and disappointment with the educational system they are the part of.

Ananda Lal in his introduction to the second volume of *Collected Plays of Mahesh Elkunchwar* exhibits the repulsive tone of the play. He says:

> *Holi* was Elkunchwar's first major play, albeit short, and surely the product of an angry young man (he was barely thirty years old) about angry young men. The play highlights the frustration of Indian students faced with a bureaucratic and authoritarian administrative system totally impervious to their needs and grievances (Lal xv).

Vijay Mehata a renowned critic and director has special consideration for the play *Holi* by Elkunchwar and she thinks as she writes in the foreword of the second volume of *Collected Plays of Mahesh Elkunchwar* that in 1970 Elkunchwar got in the mainstream of theatre with his two one-act plays *Sultan* and *Holi*. He was very young then. She continues writing that "[F]rom Mahesh's earlier writings, *Holi* went on to become – and still remains-the most path-breaking experiment on many counts. It captured the restlessness and tragic frustration of students on a campus, an experience deeply felt by Mahesh as a young lecturer in Nagpur University" (Mehta xi).

Both Vijaya Mehta and Anand Lal have attempted a connection of an autobiographical nature behind the inspiration for writing the play *Holi*. However there are two different things they talk about the same person. Though Vijaya says that Mahesh was a young man then, she believes that it is his experience as teacher in Nagpur University when he saw the frustrating experiences of students. Anand Lal however thinks that the play was a result of the suppressed anger of youth of India, who wants to eradicate the bureaucratic authoritative system and it is the outcome of the wish according to which such responses must be registered; they should get voiced.

Right from the opening scene of the play, we experience the violent and angry responses by the group of students. They exhibit such tendency though the particular use of sexually abusive language, verbal attack, impatient conclusions, pessimism, repulsive tendency and violence.

When Gopal hears from Madhav that only their college does not have holiday that day, he expresses his anger. He says, "Bloody pimps go on reducing our holidays. Has even this Principal's father ever seen a holiday for *Holi* curtailed" (Elkunchwar 03). The compulsory attendance to the lecture made by the principal irritates them. Timur ironically makes fun of the person who has been declared as an 'authority' on the subject. He says, "Authority means some pseudo-scholar sermonizing on how great our Indian culture is and how you youngsters of today ought to substitute your jeans for *dhotis*!" (Elkunchwar 6)

Thakur doesn't like the way Timur talks about the hypocrisy of the speaker who declares themselves an authority in the subject. Thankur thinks that one has to study and practice things to get command over the subject and Gopal does nothing of it. Vasanta gets angry and replies to Thakur:

> Fuck off you proper speaker, you! I'll tell you what's culture. Yuou bastards making shaven widows pregnant, how dare you holler about culture? Out! Out with a fucking smoke! (Elkunchwar 6)

Exhibition of sexuality has been one of the ways of the indicators of the repulsive tendencies. The use of sexually abusive language is not aimed at only attacking the other person but it aims at achieving certain desired effects. It challenges the sexual potency of a person, which in a complex way is ambiguous and full of uncertainty of its meaning and nature. However there exists a lifelong confusion and doubt about the sexual capability and strength in one's mind especially before one gets acquainted with sexual experience. It is here the sexual fantasies play an important role. It has been the result of sum of the culturally constructed ideas of sexuality i.e. manliness or feminine.

When Foucault says in his book *The History of Sexuality: An Introduction* that 'silence' has been assigned a significant role to play as far as the expression of sexuality is concerned. He presents whole network of reasons and discourse in the particular historical period when such silence was maintained and sometimes free expression was also sought on a certain standpoints. This issue however in Indian context holds significance on various levels perhaps since the gravity of the silence in this context is more severe than Foucault might have experienced in different spacio-temporal context. He observes a similar thing about the classical age. He says,

> We are informed that if repression has indeed been the fundamental link between power, knowledge, and sexuality since the classical age, it stands to reason that we will not be able to free ourselves from it except at a considerable cost: nothing less than a transgression of laws, a lifting of prohibitions, an irruption of speech, are instating of pleasure within reality, and a whole new economy in the mechanisms of power will be required. For the least glimmer of truth is conditioned by politics (Foucault 05).

It is almost in all the cultures, the abusive sexual expressions are visible. It is also evident that the more political turmoil the country faces, the more the youth of the country develops repulsive tendencies. It is Vasanta's remark about sexual experience he had, makes the idea of sexual expression an important one. After the discussion on the need of 'grown hair down there' for being able to make love, Vasanta does not miss the opportunity in showing his knowledge of sexual experience. He says:

> Why do you need hair for making love? I had made love in my effing seventh standard. The flogging I'd got from my father, darling! How was I to know the effing fossil was watching from a hole in the door? (Elkunchwar 07)

His remark suggests two things. First his expression on the issue psychologically sets him free at least on the basis of showing and being able to show his knowledge and ability of making love in his seventh standard and secondly his anger against his father's dominance. The discussion over the importance of cow urine ultimately leads to dig out the dire disappointment of the youth on the campus. Vasanta replies to Timur:

> So has human piss! Wanna drink it? Bastard, if one person drinks it, you pseudo-culturist think it's piss, but if all drink, then what's it? Elixir of life! Bravo! Culture! On one hand, we have these effing culturists and on the other, those khaddar-wearing freaks! Fuckers have completely fucked up our lives. Out with a smoke! (Elkunchwar 13)

With this remark of Vasanta the disappointment becomes very clear. It is also indicative of the variety of issues that ultimately hatch the repulsive tendencies of youth. Vasanta's attack on the 'culturists' is actually on the tendency that unnecessarily gives importance to the trivial things. There are many activities a society has to perform though they are not important or necessary. And it becomes the target of attack when the movement begins to bring about the change in the thinking that is based on blind beliefs. In Indian context, complexity of the problem grows larger than life due to many reasons. The major concern in this regard is the ignorance of the meaning of culture and the necessity of its preservation especially in the times when foreign cultures are intruding. The citizens of a nation always possess a tendency and concern for preservation for their culture that has been brought to them in the form of history, monuments, songs, folklore, literature and tales in oral traditions. Every strata of the nation however possesses it in different ways with all its variety at the level of age, religion, caste, region, history, gender, role, class, etc. Here in the play *Party*, it is mainly the youth who attacks the two important issues of Indian social consciousness. The first is culture that creates and sustains a typical thinking and the second it is the politics that affects larger part of the social life. The disappointment of Ranjit is revealed through his remark about the politicians and businessmen. He says:

> I have just one effing ambition. Collect some potbellied ministers, some fat businessmen, and removing their clothes in some public square, kick them on their naked asses! (Elkunchwar 13)

Gopal says that there should be one correction in Ranjit's remark that after they are done with the kicking, they should set rabid dogs after them. The intensity of the revolt is felt only with the timely growth of the repulsive responses from majority of sections from a society. Generally it takes a considerable time to bring about such kind of unification of responses. It requires many things till it comes to the terms of collective response. Until it happens, the society and the sections in the society experience many small revolts. It does not become necessary always that it should be accompanied by violence or the visibility of the change as an aftermath of the revolt. Every effort of resistance and of showing aggression matters in the process of building a response that ultimately contributes to the thought that becomes the base of a revolution. Murray N. Rothbard in his book *Eagalitarianism as a Revolt Against Nature and other Essays* defines the word 'revolution' in a specific larger manner. He writes about common opinions about revolution which are mainly manufactured by media and virtual reality. Explains the nature of revolution and says:

> Revolution is a mighty, complex, long-run process, a complicated movement with many vital parts and functions. It is the pamphleteer writing in his study; it is the journalist, the political club, the agitator, the organizer, the campus activist, the theoretician, the philanthropist. It is all this and much more. Each person and group has its part to play in this great complex movement (Rothbard 191).

Before the denouement of the play comes with the lighting up the fire of *Holi*, suicide of Anand and appearance of police on the stage for interrogation, one could feel the presence of the evidences of feelings of revolt in different forms. The treatment they give to Anand is an outcome of the anger they have harbored against the system. Unfortunately Anand becomes the victim of it. But the treatment is an evidence of the violent capability the youth has developed in the years. When Vasanta expresses his anger in the following statement:

> I've seen so many culture-wallahs really need to be praised. Build temples and gobble up the money.

Spouting religious shit all the while. Who's that
Desaiji coming today? Supposed to be blessed one.
Keep looting bastards, in the name of god, religion,
and the nation! You bloody Brahmins have fucked up
everything! (Elkunchwar 14)

It becomes more obvious of its multifaceted nature of
repulsive tendencies the youth on the campus has developed.
Vasanta supposes Brahmins are responsible for bringing in
the redundancy of culture in Indian society. Politics, business,
education system, *varna* system, cultural teaching have turned
antagonistic to the students and it represents on the larger
scale the Indian situation in which the youth of India vainly
attempts to come over them. The multitude of the issues has
one of the major concerns. It eventually reduces them to the
thinking of impossibility of any change. It also results in losing
one's faith in the possibility of a change in lawful and gradual
manner. It poses the challenges to the positive attitude by
which possibility of desired change is sought on the basis of
truth, rights, appropriateness, justice and non-violence.

The inevitability of revolt by the youth is strengthened
by the way the forces that straightway affect and disturb the
youth in a dominant manner. The discourse of power always
looks after its sustenance and security. There are always two
ways to bring about a change in any system. One is internally
and the second is externally. One can bring changes in a system
by becoming the part of it. When it is not possible to become
the part of the system, the revolt becomes necessary to turn
it topsy-turvy. But the superstructure does not however allow
the possibility of revolt. The knowledge of this again turns the
youth to despair. It is the reason why Ranjit says that he "feels
like burning all the fucking buildings down!" (Elkunchwar
20). The treatment they give to Anand as punishment for
revealing their names to the Principal or lighting up *Holi*

fire by using the chair from the hostel recreation room has been symbolic of the revolt the students wish to bring out against the all the adverse conditions they wish to change and annihilate the evil practices of the system they cannot change.

It appears that the inevitability of revolt does exist not only in the public and external spheres with all its political and social implications but personal dimensions do have their roles in it. Sexually abusive language suggests the anger of the youth and the abusive terminology imply deeply the problematic of sexuality and questions the notions of various sexual orientations. In *Autobiography*, we get to witness the revolt of a woman that has been instigated by certain personal tendencies developed in the course of time. Unlike the political implication for the repulsive tendencies developed by the youth in *Holi and Autobiography* presents a way to suggest how there exits another possibility of repulsive attitude that could result into a revolt on the small scale. Unlike the revolt against the totalitarianism prevailing as a part of whole system as felt by the students in the college in *Holi*, *Autobiography* offers an opportunity to consider the development of problematic of the culminations of the action one decides to take in order to activate the revolt against the influence, power, helplessness and lack of identity.

Though here in *Autobiography* it is Vasanti who seeks revenge on her elder sister Uttara for the bad treatment she receives from her. It is not the only cause that Uttara never identified her younger sister as worth human being but it is Uttara's overall behavior that changed after marriage brought the sense of anger in Vasanti. The unfair practice of elder sister to keep her younger sister under control and exhibiting frequently the patronizing gesture towards her harbors in her the feeling of revolt that ultimately succeeds in confiscating the reason of Uttara's vanity. It is how Vasanti planned. What becomes of it is altogether a different story. But the question remains how such type of antagonism is constructed and what its ingredients are.

Sexuality and realization of sexual powers in a social context occur on two level of gender crudely one a female realizing or subjugating her female sexual identity under male dominance and social structure of institutions and roles of a female in them and the certain family system.

In *Party* Elkunchawar seems to be putting the event of party and the exhibition of a group of certain people enjoying a status in society away from the painful experiences and labor of life, as the preface for the situation when an activist like Amrit is killed. After independence India has witnessed few movements which consisted of revolutionary ideas both socially and politically. Few of them chose violent ways to attain their goal while others trusted law and order and thought the democratic ways would bring them help. Dalit movement had to go through the ways where violence and atrocities were frequently faced and its history has not remained homogeneous. It is also certain that a situation guarantees the revolt in which a point is reached where injustice is so high that it gets unbearable, slave like and all possible ways of hopeful life are shut. *Adivasi* people in India have been triply subjugated and the growing vicious impact of capitalism is making their live impossible by denying them their freedom to live independently relying on natural resources and even destroying the resources in terms of profit.

Agashe, Bharat and Barve belong to the community of writers and are enjoying a party given by Damayanti in honour of Barve for getting an award. Their talk brings the idea of a world where they have no connection of the life the common people live; their only concerns remain around the personal development in terms of awards, money and foreign tours. It all happens under the false pretense of creativity and understanding of life. The news of death of Amrit brings them a shock. Though there had been talk that the reason for Amrit's going to tribal region and fighting for their rights is his frustration and disappointment in love but it is Doctor who tells Damyanti in the beginning of the play that she should not mix idealism up with romanticism. He says:

> Actually Amrit isn't even an idealist. He's convinced that many people in our society are exploited with nobody on their side to fight. So he's gone across-that's all. As simple and straightforward as that, the way he sees it (Elkunchwar 159).

It is Doctor who is a 'spectator watching the glittering world' asserts the division of the society in terms of this side and going across the side. It is always expected that a nation should never be oblivious to the painful patches it has developed or developing. Since the complexity of the various factors that contribute in making a nation great and flawless, grows with the presence of variety of discrimination in time, space and culture of people. Strangeness of the situation grows more vivid with the nature of the struggle. Some people like Mohini are not able to sleep because they are pestered by the idea that they are not loved anymore and consumption of alcohol does not help them either whereas the people in the tribal areas are living a life worse than animals. They do not even get sufficient food to eat; clothes to cover their bodies, primary education to their children and basic aids if they fall ill. It is way far away from the phrases like right to education, right to information, right to live, freedom of speech and it is the reason the ignorance do not even bring them idea that they have the right to fight it back. The fatalistic ideas prevail the regions so deep psychologically and it plays a vital role in bringing hurdles in the ways of new ideas of development.

Simultaneously a larger part of the society remains oblivious and ignorant to the plights of the people living so miserable life. It is with a sort of adventure of few truly learned people, attempts are made to fight against the Government and the prevailing systems that do not allow any change that challenges their advantageous positions. It is the reason why Amrit is killed who organized the *adivasis* and did demonstration there. The journalist Jogdand talks about the dramatic show of the power of state through the police and military organization. It is how the very system that has been created to protect the people of a nation against injustice, operates to sustain and take care of the advantage and benefits of certain people that hold the main streams of power including itself. He says:

> The armed police have been posted there for the last fifteen days. On adivasi lands. Amrit's been taking out demonstrations of hundreds. A stone hurled from somewhere hits a policeman. Then there is a lathi charge. Then teargas shells. A show of rifles. Very dramatic. Very very dramatic (Elkunchwar 187).

It is only Jogdand who brings the information to the people at the party how the government wants to give license and facilities to a couple of big promoters so that they can deforest the entire area and once the land is developed the prices around the area will shoot up and the land is owned by the wife of the chief minister. As Barve talks to Damyanti he makes the idea clear how there has been hypocrisy in his writing that boast of writing noble human feelings based on experience. He tells her the incident when he was going to Delhi to receive the award. It is there he realizes poverty prevailing in the country when he sees poor women and children standing in the rain. He confesses that:

> I could see no relation any longer between my words
> and the agony of the endless suffering of these people.
> My words are no words. They are like an outer skin
> that can be discarded. Amrit knew this. That is
> what made me feel uncomfortable in his presence.
> May be Amrit had realized this when he went away
> (Elkunchwar 197).

The discussion at the party is clearly indicative of the several Indias that exist devoid of the knowledge of each other though they are related to the core with each other internally but they do not realize the connection nor do they wish to acquire knowledge of it. It eventually brings about the widening of the distance between the two areas. With the growth of time it fortifies the stability of the conditions and brings about the impossibility of changing it. It is not affected only politically and economically but the impact of the differences and inequalities go down deep into the psychological, cultural, ethnic and traditional spaces.

In the novel *The White Tiger* by Arvind Adiga the protagonist Balram Halwai writes to Jiabao the difference between the two Indias: the choice. According to him in cities one can remain good if one chooses to be so but in villages there is no choice. Lack of choice to be good or remain good is denial to get knowledge or rather sustenance of ignorance. It is the perpetuation of criminal traditions through exploitative and oppressive regime. Political, social, economical and moral developments seem to be positive for such regime to continue as they are the results of it or vice versa. It becomes no matter of wonder to see democracy and village people discussing the elections "like eunuchs discussing the *Kamasutra*" (Adiga 98).

Amrit knew what he was doing would not bring a revolution but it is the way he had chosen to bring justice to the people in the region. His has been a non violent way of struggling for the rights of the tribal. But it is also true as Balram says there is no choice in villages to remain good for everyone. He wronged the many institutions and giants who held the power and were reluctant to release the hold of them on it. It certainly connects to the movement that began in the small village in West Bengal called Naxalbari. It then very notoriously developed itself making violence its main tool to affect the state regime and control. The base of the movement however was the atrocities and injustice the tribal have been facing since and before of colonization. It is also notable to realize the situation when India dreams of becoming world power and at the same time it has certain areas of darkness where ignorance about such dreams prevails.

It is more than half century since India received freedom from British rule and larger part of the population of India cannot conceive what exactly it means to be free. The glory of freedom and the national consciousness have gradually ebbed away and large poverty ridden section of the society realized that there will be no 'avatar' that can bring changes in their lives. It was not only the unruly rule of the British Government that had vicious impact on Indian life. But during the shift of power from the 'anarchical' regional rule of the kings to the control of the landlords over the means of production, the oppressed never received any opportunity of progression. As a consequence, various means were attempted to deal with the vicious circles poverty has created. Violence was one of the most prominent of them. Of course one must never forget that it is the last weapon one has to choose realizing well the possible threat to one's existence. Naxalbari was the first village to embark upon the violent act towards 'freedom'.

Though there have been vast developments in the movement, reducing it to more ideological complexity, this 'people's war' does not seem to lose its grounds since they are buried in their age long poor conditions and humiliation. The changing nature of economy has brought but more disheartening and challenging conditions making their lives impossible and state's totalitarian regime poses political impossibility. In his article *in Economical and Political Weekly* in August 1972 Mohan Ram emphasized,

> [W]ith the arrest of Charu Muzumdar, just as five years ago they gleefully pronounced revolution in India dead with failure of the Naxalbari up-rising, as though Naxalbari was the beginning and end of the Indian revolution. It was neither; at best it could be vested with a certain symbolism (Ram 1471).

This transformation from non-violence to violence is an upshot of so many contradicting and antithetical thoughts rising in his minds. The realization of helplessness and humiliation as a reward for the money brings out the feelings. On the other hand, holding on factual line of recent development in Naxal crises in November 2008 PCAPA (People's Committee Against Police Atrocities) led mass protest against police brutality. The spokespersons of PCAPA Asit Mahato declared the outfit would no longer continue democratic protest. "After continuous torture by the joint forces, the PCAPA has decided to combat the forces" (Mittal 30). The bureaucrats sitting at capital repeat the much void statement:

> However the depth of the fear imbedded in such statements provides us with the revolutionary potentials that exist in the country. Indian mindset requires breaking through the shackles of human civilization oscillates between the 'Freedom from Fear' and the 'Fear of Freedom'… The contest may be physical, existential, political and social. Freedom without context is too abstract to contemplate (Mohanty 220).

In the end of the play all characters leave the party place and move to their places with certain gestures after hearing the news of murder of Amrit. The dramatist is successful in showing the typical nature of various psychologies dominant in the society especially those representing middle class which is self indulgent. It is no wonder how certain type of people have such crude and false fantasies for the very sensitive issues in the society. But the choice the people like Amrit make are not out of romanticism but it is the faithful activism that believes for a better change.

It seems that the treatment Elkunchwar gives to the subject matter of revolutionary ideas of both scale smaller and larger can be divided in two ways. The revolt his characters bring about in the certain form is social and political. It could further be divided into tiny segment of social and political nature. Secondly he has strength in depicting the revolt on personal and psychological level. It is of course also true that mingling and complex nature and presence of different characteristics of personal, social, cultural, political and psychological issues in the plays does not allow to divide them into tight categories. It is however easier to realize the strong current of the predominant issue.

In *Garbo, Party, Desire in the Rocks, As One Descardeth the Old Clothes..., Reflection, Autobiography,* there exists the acts of revolution especially by the female characters that could be called as what Kate Millett in her book *Sexual Politics* called it as 'sexual revolution'. Garbo in *Garbo*, Lalita in *Desire in the Rocks*, Aai in *As One Descardeth the Old Clothes...*, woman in *Reflection* and Vasudha in *Autobiography* do possess certain aura of the sexual revolution. Their major concern however seems to be acting against the patriarchal forces that have been keeping them in submissive gestures. It is important to recognize how patriarchy and construction sexuality and female identity have been effective naturalizing the artificial category of the feminine.

It has taken years for women to be recognized as human beings and they too deserve the rights of every kind being the important part of society as men are. Women have undergone the trauma of suffering of manifold. They have been doubly suppressed being female that has to be feminine and woman who is 'other' in male dominated society. It takes just a moment of realization against the suppression for a revolt. Women come to realization in a specific situation and conflict the agencies through which they have been dominated and the dominance have been naturalized. It takes more time, more degree of suffering and realization of vanity and meaninglessness of certain cultural construction and practices. Strange enough, in the situation of such realization women tend to react in a manner which is also a result of patriarchal system. The actions of resistance also seem to be defined and maintained for or against patriarchal discourses. The possibility of erasing the inevitability of the conflict between the binary opposition appears less. It mainly happens due to the nature of cultural creations and process of significance.

In her book *Sexual Politics* Kate Millette divides the revolution in two phases Sexual Revolution first phase 1830 -1930 and the Counter Revolution 1930 -1960. She studies it in terms of politics, literature, reactionary policy and ideology. She writes;

> A sexual revolution would require... an end of traditional sexual inhibition and taboos, particularly those that most threatens patriarchal monogamous marriage: homo-sexuality, "illegitimacy", adolescent, pre- and extra-marital sexuality. The negative aura with which sexual activity has generally been surrounded would necessarily be eliminated, together with the double standard and prostitution. (Milllett 62).

With this Millett thinks that the event of revolution would have certain characteristics like 'permissive single standard of sexual freedom,' and it is 'uncorrupted by the crass and exploitative economic bases of traditional sexual alliances'.

In *Garbo*, Garbo is murdered by the trio who represent the forces of patriarchy in society. They could be in the form of intellectual, richness and fancy. It is how the trio represents their significance being male to the female Garbo. Before Garbo is killed, it makes an intelligible show of functioning of matriarchal subjugation against Garbo and she has been the victim of the double standards of sexuality as Millett calls it.

Society looks down upon the prostitutes and considers it evil relating it with characteristically bad nature of the prostitutes. Society does not recognize the complete lack of choice for the prostitutes and it is the society which does not offer any way out. The situation where patriarchal conditions already closes off the ways through which economic stability could be sought by women, becomes responsible to refrain them from resistance and attack the system. Garbo has to work as junior artist in order to earn money for her livelihood. For it she requires to be fit and look beautiful. Her pregnancy becomes threat for her career as an artist and she knows that a life as a wife to rear the child is impossible for her due to the label of prostitute. She accepts and knows it well what value she holds in society.

The trio knows her body and receives different meaning of the relationship they have developed with her. The peculiarity of their thought is that they consider her only the 'other' in making their opinion regarding her. Shrimant says: "Her (Garbo's) only business in life has been jumping from bed to bed. She's nothing but a sex-machine" (Elkunchwar 16). Shrimant reduces her to inanimate mechanical object. She has been denied of value being human. Though Shrimant says that she is great in bed, she remains only a sex machine for him. Though he recognizes goodness in her, it has been Garbo status being woman and a prostitute both does offer him to think that she is just a commodity to be paid for and consumed. Intuc on the other hand philosophizes her value in his own way. He says that the idea that woman is an enigma is not true. He considers it a kind of literary stupidity. It is here he confesses how a woman is cheaply treated every time. She remains an attraction until the time she is not explore (sexually). Once it happens, she loses her importance in the mind of the male. Intuc expects:

> A woman should be able to satisfy you fully, and yet withhold a part of herself from you … To put it in a nutshell, Garbo never becomes common. Even after fulfilling the needs of all three of us, a part of her still remains untouched (G 18-19).

Garbo is pregnant and she tries to tell the trio about her pregnancy but every one of them makes fun of her. In the talk she realizes more how it is impossible to think of motherhood for her. Though it is the child of Intuc, the trio is afraid that she would plant it on one of them. Intuc asks Shrimat:

> And why the hell did she get into this messy situation when mother hood is the easiest thing to avoid these days? It can't be the first time it's happened to her. Why come here and tell us about it? Do you think she's going to plant this on one of us? (Elkunchwar 35)

It is this realization that brings Garbo to the terms of killing the child in her womb. It is not that she straightway decided to kill the child. She wanted to give birth to the child but she knew what worse kind of fate would trouble the fatherless child. She never intends to tell them whose child she was bearing nor wanted them to take the responsibility of the child as a father. She expects form them they should help her in this by taking the responsibility being friends of hers. It should never matter who the father of the child was. She also realizes and expresses that the minute she becomes pregnant, she also becomes cheap. She rather sarcastically mentions how they followed her like dogs. She tells them that she did not come to them to have sympathy or help; she just came there as she was feeling lonely. However she declares that;

> But today I've seen you in your true colour. Remember one thing though I could not implicate all three of you in this if I wanted to, so don't think you can shrug off responsibility (Elkunchwar 36).

She had been for a period of time under the influence of Intuc's romanticism and she admits that it brought her dreams to live a happy life as a woman should deserve. She tells Intuc that it is not so easy to remain in that sheer romanticism. Her mind became so calculating with the pressure of the life that has to be lived with the help of money and for money one has to struggle when the person is a woman. She realizes though she feels tenderness for someone for certain times, her mind gives the intimations about the dangers of such development and lack of life for such relationship. She knows the hardship the attachment would follow. Though Intuc, Pansy and Shrimant attempt hard to convince her that they would be people who will take care of her child and give name to it but she knows the impossibility besides the damage it would bring to her livelihood as she will not be able to work anymore and would lose everything eventually.

Gabo's becomes the revolt against the social conditions when all doors are shut for a gender and set of people who have been caught in a structure of values and relations. Garbo is to certain degree successful in bringing a kind of assertion of independence through the way she utilizes her body for personal gains. She becomes a powerful woman with the magic of her sexual gesture. She too knows that it brings her authority of revolt against the society that does not allow her an easy life.

No revolt however is devoid of pain, suffering and sacrifice. It is done with much labour. The pain for Garbo is in taking decision to kill her child in her womb keeping aside all the longing for motherhood. She thought at least the director would have a pale face when he realizes that she had abortion but she finds there no one except a huge, coarse woman. Her suffering ends with her murder by Shrimant who does not wish to allow her to leave the place. She could have been a woman for him who would guarantee the world about his potency and masculinity. When she does not respond to him, he kills her. It is how she keeps on becoming the victim of almost every kind of difficulties the patriarchy and subjugation of women. It gets over with her murder only.

In *Desire in the Rocks* Lalita comes to terms with suicidal thought and succeeds in it due to certain realization that have been brought to her by understanding consisting of discovery of nature of love her brother has for her. It has been so due to the destruction of the conceptions on which she had been constructed her philosophy of life. It mainly consisted of the ideas of love that crossed the boundaries of kinship and the thought they were doing something wrong hardly touched since Hemkant was the only savior for her after the traumatic period of time she experienced when her father Dadasaheb was alive and after the death of her father, the trustees troubled her. Lalita lived a lonely life in the huge mansion of them. She grew so dependent on her brother Hemkant that she would never bear the thought of Hemkant going way from her.

There were several patterns that made Lalita behave in suicidal way. The death of her mother, brother becoming rebellious against father and leaving the home, father's negligence towards her, father's strict nature, her everlasting loneliness, have been the key factors that made her weak at core of her heart. She being a child could not cope up with it and developed a liking towards her brother. It was mainly in pursuit of love that she never received. She surrenders herself to Hemkant and she knows it. She says:

> Don't. Don't you come near me. Brute. You know I'm weak. And so full of yearning. Hem, even if you don't come to me, I will. I'll follow you wherever you go. Like a shadow. Hem. How am I? (Elkunchwar 89)

Though there has been the moment when she feels that she has been getting the love she longs for. When Hemkant tells her that she is beautiful, she says him to say that again and she "can give him anything to hear this over and over again". (Elkunchwar 91). Intensity has been major characteristics of her passion for Hemkant. Hemkant takes her to old mansion in the village full of rocks so that he can carve statues there. He is so engrossed in his work that he spends more time in that work. On the other hand, Lalita is afraid of darkness and loneliness but becomes ready to live with Hemkant there since she cannot live without him. It is only with the realization that Hemkant has messed up the idea of love with the idea of art and its permanence. Hemkant does know that Lalita is too weak to dare to think independently and realize that he is leaving no space for her to exist independently. Lalita expresses her conditions truly. She says:

> I am your slave. Oh Lord, my lord. When you descend from there, I will spread my hair under you feet. Trample over me. The seal of your authority has been stamped on every drop of my blood. My body is yours,

my heart is yours, my will is yours. I am nothing but
a pile of dried leaves without you; a mere sapless plant
trailing on the ground. One glance from your eyes
and I sprout tender green leaves. You blow life into
my body with just your voice, your glance, your touch
(Elkunchwar 95-6).

Lalita eventully realizes that Hemkant values his work more
than her love and her pregnancy. She begs to him to be with
her because she needs him at that time but Hemkant does not
realize the importance of it. She tells Hemkant how there is a
void in the idea of art he has. She tells him that he does not even
understand the idea of creation and he cannot be a creator. It is
because she thinks that creation is a very easy thing and one has
to realize it being human. For her Hemkant is no human. She
loses her child and realizes the curse that had been effective in
the mansion. She revolts against him. It has indeed been against
the attitude that considers humanity lesser than anything else.
Though it is not a revolt that aims at challenging a patriarchal
or masculine world that does activate its holds for sustenance
of its power. It is the revolt of an innocent and devoted mind
against the ruthlessness and numbness of human mind lacking
human feeling. The realization that Hemkant does not love her
as she imagined him doing so makes her lose faith over her love
for him. He was the only man for whom she fought against the
whole world. The strength she received for it was from the idea
that the love they were in had been pure and she trusted him
a true lover and artist. When she comes to know that he has
given the child to the beggar to bury, her faith gets destructed
completely. It is then she grows repulsive. The idea that she has
sinned becomes dominant in her mind. She says:

It's like a patch of leukoderma that has spread all over
the whole body. A few days of shame, but when the

whole body is covered, what shame can there be? Sin
once. Then it's over that's not how it is. Sin never ends
(Elkunchwar 115).

Lalita goes in search of salvation from the sin. She becomes
an independent person after experiencing the great pain. She
wanders the places so that she could get rid of the feelings of
sin. She brings pains to her body. She expects her body to fall
but it does not happen. She says:

> I am inflicting this on myself. I have sinned. Mustn't
> I be judged? I am going to burn myself. In his fire of
> retribution, Hem. I want to be pure again. Hem, I have
> laid this body under so many bodies. As retribution.
> Even them my heart won't stop breaking. Why doesn't
> it stop? Hem, hem, the retribution for sin is to remain
> in sin forever. To continue sin (Elunchwar 124).

Hemkant was responsible in bringing about the destruction
of Lalita and himself. Lalita's only fault was that she loved
him and trusted love for love's sake. Hemknat observed only
objective reality and could never learn and reach the pure light
of truth. He brought the layers of feeling on the outer parts of
the stones but he could never reach the realty of feeling and
human desire. He could not understand the truth in the centre
of reality. Lalita went through the ordeals of the reality and
pain. The major reasons for her transformation from Lalita
who was fearful and needful of protection, to the person who
was fearless, self negating and emotionally neutral were the
destruction of the emotional and ideal world where Hemkant
was a considerate human being. The realization of Hemkant's
true nature instigates Lalita to become repulsive and lose her
faith, child, and life including that of Hemkant.

Works Cited

Adiga, Arvind. *The White Tiger.* New Delhi: Harper Collins, 2008. Print.

Chakroborty, Kaustav, ed. *Indian Drama in English.* New Delhi: PHI Learning Pvt. Ltd., 2011. Print.

Elkunchwar, Mahesh. *Collected Plays of Mahesh Elkunchwar Vol. I.* New Delhi: Oxford University Press, 2009. Print.

Elkunchwar, Mahesh. *Collected Plays of Mahesh Elkunchwar Vol. II.* New Delhi: Oxford University Press, 2011. Print.

Foucault, Michael. *The History of Sexuality. Vol. I.* New York: Vintage Books. 1990. Print.

Hobsbawm, Eric. *The Age of Revolution 1789 – 1848.* New York: Vintage Books. 1996. Print.

Lal, Madan. Introduction. *Collected Plays of Mahesh Elkunchwar Vol. II.* New Delhi: (2011): xxii. Print.

Mathi, Nirai.S. "Mahashweta Devi, the Rebel Playwright of Mother of 1084." *The Literary Criterion* 3&4 (2007): 33. Print.

Mehta, Vijaya. Foreword. *Collected Plays of Mahesh Elkunchwar Vol. I.* By Elkunchwar. New Delhi: Oxford University Press. 2011. Print.

Millette, Kate. *Sexual Politics.* Urbana and Chicago: University of Illinois Press, 1970. Print.

Mittal, Tusha. "How a Deaf Ear is Turning Plughshares to Swords". *Tehelka* 44 (2009): 30. Print.

Mohanty, Prafull. K. "Freedom as Identity: The Literature of Rising". *Indian Literature, Sahitya Akademi's Bi-Monthly Journal* 1. (2009): 220. Print.

Ram, Mohan, "Five Years After Naxalbari." *Economic and Political Weekly* 7 Web (1972): 1471.

Pendhari, Supriya. *Marathi Natyasrushtitil Vidroh ani Navata.* Nagpur: Vijay Prakashan, 2002. Print.

Rothbard, Murray N. *Eagalitarianism as a Revolt Against Nature and Other Essays.* Auburn: 2000. Print.

Salunkhe. A.H. *Astikshiromani: Charvak.* Satara: Lokayat Prakashan, 1992. Print.

Zizek, Slavoj. *The Plague of Fantsies.* London: Verso, 1997. Print.

Chapter IV
'VIOLENCE' IN THE SELECT PLAYS OF MAHESH ELKUNCHWAR

Violence is one of the vital issues Elkunchwar seems to give special treatment in his plays. Unlike Tendulkar, Elkunchwar does not offer more explicit space to violence. However violence appears at juncture when it is sought as the culmination and outcome of crisis of conflict of human issues. Ending of the plays like *Desire in the Rocks, Garbo, Sultan, Party, Holi,* are violent nature. Violence takes place in the plays in the form of murder, suicide, torture, humiliation, etc.

In this chapter attempts are made to examine the depiction of violent acts of the characters in the plays in two ways. The first way is to evaluate the performance of the violence on the stage and its impact on the audience. The mechanism and the scheme of presentation of the violence on the stage have a significant role to play in Elkunchwar's plays. Secondly the analysis of the cruelty enacted by the characters is to be sought in contextual references. The violence exhibited in the plays has its relation with sociological, psychological, cultural background of the characters.

Violence or cruelty has been recurring theme of theatrical performance. Aggression in the human behavior is considered as integral part of animal instinct. Man is a social and cultured animal. Theatre becomes an effective medium to express certain nature of social life in directed form characterized by the typical language and unities. Theatrical performances of the issues like desire, love, politics, envy, conflict, natural disaster, marital relationships, jealousy, poverty, struggle, friendship, etc have proved very effective in Marathi theatres especially in the plays of Satish Alekar, Vijay Tendulkar and Khanolkar. The theatre in the strong sense is a medium that presents a view of life in its miniature and sometimes in its magnanimous form. In forward to the book *Theatre and Violence* Catherine Cusack says,

> It seems to me that drama always had to reflect the violent forging of our world. And the refinement and changes in presentation of that violence in theatre continue to keep pace with the kinds of violence we inflict upon one another. Whether it's subtle struggle within a family, dressed-up corporate violence or state-funded annihilation (Cusack xii).

Catherine believes in the idea that violence not only seeks its revelation in ever changing forms but it necessarily possesses a quality to appear in new forms. It is not easy to state how solely drama indulges in presenting or keeping pace with the kinds of violence we inflict. It however becomes an important phenomenon to observe how drama does offer certain effects on its readers and audience crossing the boundaries of mere presentation of facts. Catherine's statement though evidently more generalized could be thought as the starting point of argument on the issue. It is so because simple act of violence that does not include large massacre or bloodshed, potentially exhibit the possibility of presence of complex and interconnected issues that instigate such acts.

Fanon in his book *The Wretched of the Earth* offers a detailed discourse on process of decolonization and violence. He deals with the issue of violence as inevitable one as far as the process of decolonization is concerned. He writes in the first chapter of the book entitled "Concerning Violence":

> National liberation, national renaissance, the restoration of nationhood to the people, commonwealth: whatever may be the headings used or the new formulas introduced, decolonization is always a violent phenomenon (Fanon 27).

In the preface of the same book Jean – Paul Sartre makes peculiar observation about the violence enacted by the colonizers. He does not take interest in the impact of the violence on colonized but mainly is concerned with the impact of violence on the colonizers. While talking about the different ways in which the old 'mother countries' exercised their power on the colonized, he offers his observation on the issue of violence enacted by the colonizers. It is no pretence on the part of Sartre to exhibit that he has no ancestral relation to the rulers. He uses the word 'we'. According to him the intensity of violence has increased many folds but there was a method in victory of the colonizers. The victories according to him did not alter them or they did not allow it to happen to them. After the violent victories, the humanism remained intact in them. But to their dismay

> [v]iolence has changed its direction… United by their profits, the peoples of the mother countries baptized their commonwealth of crimes, calling them fraternity and love; today violence, blocked everywhere, comes back on us through our soldiers, comes inside and takes possession of us… Yet our lobes seem to be in perfect condition; is it not rather the case that, since we cannot crush the natives, violence come back on its tracks, accumulates in the very depths of our nature seeks a way out? (Sartre 23,24)

Sartre however brings up a new dimension to the enquiry into the human violence. To him violence does possess the tendency to find control over the mind of human beings. It tends to act on its own. It will not be difficult to find the evidence in various folk tales and many modern stories about the longings and cravings for supernatural powers and consequently possessing them. It also becomes bigger part of the struggle of their life making them to control the powers rather than they being controlled by them. This phenomenon could be considered as a small part of the entire complex structure of the discourse of violence as it could be seen in two ways as violence being the independent agent that influences human minds and possessing the ability to exist on its own seeking the process of naturalization in the humans. Such transformation usually informed to become the characteristics of a particular sects or tribes as though it is a tendency inherited by the generation by their fore fathers. Secondly violence could be seen as an integral part of human psyche being one of the 'basic instincts'. In the case of Sartre's statement in the preface, it could be said that it is just an attempt on the part of him to exhibit especially in the context of Algerian war inevitability and 'innocence' of war when he says, "When we were victorious we practiced it without its (violence) seeming to alter us; it broke down the other, but for us men our humanism remained intact" (Satre 23).

It is also sure it was not stated in favour of the tendency by Sartre. He concludes his much sarcastic preface with the following way.

> Thus the day of magicians and fetishes will end; you will have to fight, or rot in concentration camps... Then, perhaps, when your back is to the wall, you will let loose at last that new violence which is raised up in you by old, oft-repeated crimes... The time is drawing near, I am sure, when we will join the ranks of those who make it (Sartre 26).

Franz Fanon too talks about the violence though concerning about only colonization and decolonization, with the gesture that of violence as an evil of necessary kind. Both Sartre and Fanon seem to be talking about violence in the same manner in case of describing one of the characteristics of violence in general. As we saw Sartre thinks that violence has its own mechanism of affect and works independently. The 8th edition of the *Oxford Advanced Learner's Dictionary* defines the word violence as "violent behaviour that is intended to hurt or kill somebody" and it also gives the second meaning as "physical or emotional force and energy" (OALD 1719). Though the meaning of the word in the dictionary contains the adjective 'violent', it makes clear that violence is any behaviour that intends to hurt or kill and comprises in its second entry of meaning the both aspects of violence i. e. physical and emotional. The dictionary gives the meaning of violence with much preoccupation of intentionality. And it is in this context Satre stresses the other aspect of violence itself.

Though Fanon has various issues to talk about the violence in the process of decolonization like that of legitimacy of violence and its necessity in getting rid of the colonizers who mainly operate their powers through the means of subjugation and suppression with the help of armed forces, he admits that violence has its peculiar impact on the colonized. He says:

> The native who decides to put the programme into practice, and to become its moving force, is ready for violence at all times. Form birth it is clear to him that this narrow world, strewn with prohibitions, can only be called in question by absolute violence (Fanon 29).

Violence is perhaps the most crucial phenomenon that made impact on the world especially in the form of colonization and decolonization. However it does not mean that violent attitudes did not exist prior to the process of colonization and decolonization. Violence was always an important tool in controlling people in order to sustain monarchy. Colonization stands differently in the history due to the peculiarity of its *modus operandi*. Colonization systematically operated violence and it left a water mark on the psychology of a community under the control of the empire. It is true as Fanon says violence is sought by the colonized as a means to offer solution on a problem and its prerequisites are the prohibitions and subjugations. This could be seen from the violence enacted by Mangal Pandey, Chafekar Brothers, Madanlal Dhingra, Bhagatsingh, Rajguru to Sukhdev in the process of decolonization though the persons are oddly and randomly selected from the Mutiny of 1857 to the event of hanging of Bhagat Singh. These incidents are considered as individual instances where violence is sought as a solution to the problem of colonization though it had been the part of the whole freedom movement instigated in the nation.

The extended discussion of this phenomenon of violence in the history of colonization becomes essential mainly due to its 'inheritance of loss' that has vivid impact on the Indians' psychology after the independence in 1947. Elkunchwar's plays describe the social pictures of Indian society in the time when the process of transition has been already activated. It is when the changes in the old joint family system are taking place along with the myriad technological advances and development of urban culture. Fanon makes it clear in the following way how the continuation of violence activated in the certain disguised form. He says:

> We have seen that this same violence, though kept very much on the surface all through the colonial period, yet turns in the void. We have also seen that it is canalized by the emotional outlets of dance and possession by spirits; we have seen how it is exhausted in fratricidal combats. Now the problem is to lay hold of this violence which is changing direction (Fanon 45).

In a thesis entitled *On the Principles of Political Violence and the Case of Anti-Fascist Action,* it is quoted that people like Engels, Trotsky, Karl Kautsky, Joh Harris, Sartre, Fanon and Andrent while attempting to offer meaning of violence in a Marxist way concentrating on the pre and post world war period. Engels ideas on violence from his *The Conditions of Working Class in England* (1841) are taken for analyses. According to Engels it is also violence one may not recognize from its obvious exhibition. When workers are reduced to the 'premature and unnatural end', it is a form of ideological violence. He takes into consideration the idea of violence which is activated, intentional and tends to exist in its micro disguised forms to the notions concluding, "Firstly, that a deontological argument against violence on the principle of "Thu shalt not kill' is not infallible to criticism. Secondly, violence does not have to be intentional to require justification" (12).

The thesis considers various aspects of violence but what connects the thread of our argument about the violence being an independent force is the later part of the above quotation from the thesis.

In his book *The Prince* Niccolo Machiavelli takes a practical position regarding the performance of violence as far as the qualities of a prince are concerned. He says that it is good for a prince to "maintain good faith and practice integrity rather than craft and deceit" (Machiavelli 67) but he admits that it is not completely true that it guarantees greatness of a prince. The experience of his time according to him shows that only those became great "who understood by cunning to circumvent the intelligence of others" (Machiavelli 67). And then he advises:

> You must know, therefore, that there are two ways of carrying on a contest; the one by law, and the other by force. The first is practiced by men, and the other by animals; and as the first is often insufficient, it becomes necessary to resort to the second (Machiavelli 67).

It is here Machiavelli seems to believe in two aspect of power. One as it is celebrated the good one and the second is the outcome of the empiricism. It is a part of his observation of the kings making use of violence in order to sustain the power. It becomes clear here that the idea of violence need not emerge always from the personal reservoir of experiences which are generally product of the time and space. They do appear and instigate the minds of people from the experience of the society in general. It becomes a common knowledge through the history available to the people.

With the growth of time, nature of society, politics and technological advancement became more complex and phenomenon like violence has to be reconsidered with more possibilities. One of the reasons for it could be the resistance of the 'other'. The distinction became clear that it is the conflict between the active and passive where subjugation is sought as an only way to perpetuate control in every form for all types of material gains. In the book *The Age of Revolution 1789 – 1848* Eric Hobsbawn writes about the violence of the time and changes taking place in the contemporary society mainly quickened by industrial revolution. He says:

> Drink was not the only sign of this demoralization. Infanticide, prostitution, suicide, and mental derangement have all been brought into relation with this social and economic cataclysm, thanks largely to the contemporary pioneering work of what we would today call social medicine. And so as both the increase in crime and that growing and often purposeless violence which was a sort of blind personal assertion against the forces threatening to engulf the passive (Hobsbawn 204).

It is strangely true that practices like prostitution in society always relate themselves to the violent responses. And it is witnessed in almost all the cultures. In this reference Hobsbawn appears to be one more Marxist emphasizing the relationship among prostitution, infanticide, suicide, etc and the social and economical aspects. Hobsbawn and most of the above mentioned thinkers look at violence as not a mere act of aggression or force. It becomes essential on our part to detect and analyze the whole mechanism that operates and ultimately leads to violence that could be categorized in various forms. It is to consider the phenomenon of violence is not a simple act of application of violent energy but its basics consist of the fundamentals of human nature in general. It is why Slovej Zizek writes in the introduction of his book *Violence:*

But we should learn to step back, to disentangle ourselves from the fascinating lure of this directly visible "subjective" violence, violence performed by clearly identifiable agent. We need to perceive the contours of the background which generates such outbursts. A step back enables us to identity a violence that sustains our every effort to fight violence and to promote tolerance (Zizek 9).

Dr. B. R. Ambedkar in his review of *Principles of Social Reconstruction* by Bertrand Russell, first published in *Journal of the Indian Economic Society*, Vol. I, 1918, offers his didactic ideas on violence. He says:

True enough that violence cannot always be avoided and non-resistance can be adopted only when it is a better way of resistance. But the responsibility for an intelligent control of force rests on us all. In short, the point is that to achieve anything we must use force: only we must use it constructively as energy and not destructively as violence (Ambedkar 06).

Elkunchwar wrote *Garbo* a tragedy in 1973. It ends with the murder of Garbo 'a petty actress in B grade movies' the trio Intuc, Shrimant and Pansy. Though what we see in the last scene of the play is a murder where Pansy accuses Garbo to be cheating the three of them and Shrimant plunging a knife into her. This violent act could be seen from at least four perspectives representing the four characters in the plays. As it is obvious from the names, they represent the attitudes in the society. At a larger level it relates with the patriarchal dominance and violence as seen is a always a means to guarantee the dominance and sustenance of the control. Intuc seems to be the only character offering deeper philosophical perspectives on life through his refined talk. In the introduction to the *Collected Plays of Mahesh Elkunchwar* Samik Bandopadhyay writes:

> The drama in Garbo grows out of a claustrophobic real-life situation pushed to the limits of endurance, burgeoning into a surreal holy dream that is too unreal and brittle to stand the test. But what gives the fantasy its compelling magnetism is the sheer power of Intuc's words, coming in waves of cynicism, disgust, self-pity, lacerating introspection, flights of sacred vision (Bandopadhyay xv).

Garbo knows that her doing the scene in the film where she would ride a camel would result in abortion. They could have used her double in the scene. She deliberately brings about the death of the foetus growing in her womb. It however is the first instance of violence in the play and the second is murder of Garbo. Feticide becomes the reason of the murder. Though Samik Bandopadhyay give more space talking on *Garbo* in his introduction, he does not offer any critique on the violence in the play.

Garbo's decision to kill the child has ideological groundings. It is only Garbo knew that it was Intuc's child. But she could never bear the idea of bringing up the child. It is because she knew it well that it was not a simple thing to bear that responsibility since it would result in losing her roles in the movies she was already doing. And thus eventually she would lose the only source of her earning. She knew it well that she was only a 'sex machine' for the trio. It was the combination of the realization what she thinks of herself, what society thinks of her and the trio thinks of her. The presence of the three views mainly affects her illusion and delusion. Human activities and thoughts are governed with ideology which actively functions in every belief and non belief. Garbo seems to be acting in a certain manner as an obvious response to the conformist society. The thoughts of Garbo that ultimately result in decisions and actions are significantly governed by her place in the society and the social structure along with the gender she represents. She is doubly suppressed. She being a woman becomes the victim of male dominated society that exercises its power on female gender to sustain its control upon it. It is not only true about the gender discrimination but also it functions similarly in case of every passive agent or the agent reduced to the passivity within a category. For the trio Garbo was not only a woman inferior to men but also a prostitute, a woman of no importance, a 'sex machine' what Shrimant would call her. Though Garbo is lured into loving Intuc and losing herself in the romantic idea of loving life, she does not however give herself to it. The ideology that sustains the control could be seen in the following remarks of Garbo as she replies Intuc:

> I will not be happy with anybody now. It is too late for all that. Too late for happiness. For love... The mind has grown too calculating. If ever I feel momentary tenderness for anybody, the mind rears its head and hisses, 'Are you in your sense? You are playing with fire. You know what suffering will follow (Elkuchwar 57).

She comes to the terms of renunciation and such kind of one's agreement with the situation does have various roots that form the whole of the gesture one assumes. She seeks the suppression of two natural sort of desires one that of becoming mother and rearing a child of her own and secondly she abandons the possibility of her happy married life or life with a partner, whom the society would not object. Her inclination towards Intuc is obvious but she does not intend to tell him that the child is his. She knows it would be a burden for him. Besides it she has already taken the decision about its abortion. Violent act in this way appears to be of two types. These are two ways of looking at the act of violence. One is that of simple kind where Garbo comes to term with the abortion. It seems to be very clear utilitarian judgment. She cannot earn her livelihood without the job she does in the B grade movies. She does not believe in any future her child would have. This first category on the superficial level does not appear in a normal social context justifiable. The act is negated telling it as an anti-humanitarian act.

Secondly it is the ideology that influences a human mind in a certain manner when an individual cannot conceive the idea of going against the established system as one is taught to believe in immortal and fortified structure of beliefs. Beliefs are certain visible part of ideological structure. Some of them are more obvious and many of them are very difficult to recognize their ideological orientation due to their naturalization. The first part of his book *Discipline and Punish* Foucault has explained his research regarding torture as form of punishment and its relation with power and knowledge. He writes:

> To analyse the political investment of the body and the microphysics of power presupposes, therefore, that one abandons – where power is concerned – the violence – ideology opposition, the metaphor of property, the model of the contract or of conquest; that – where knowledge is concerned – one abandons the opposition between what is 'interested' and what is 'disinterested', the model of knowledge and the primacy of the subject (Foucault 28).

It is here in the light of Foucault's remark, this phenomenon of abortion of the child and the murder of Garbo by the trio could be understood with certain differences. The violence in the both the cases has the form of 'crime and punishment'. Garbo chooses the abortion instead of the violation of social norms that do not expect a 'cheap woman', a prostitute to rear a child. Secondly this violent act could be performed in a secret manner where there would be no question of identification and economic conditions were the pretext for her to rely on.

On the other hand, Garbo posed challenge to the power of the trio on the different personal levels of them. They had no problem with the conditions as long as she was giving them the physical pleasure being a 'sex machine'. For Pansy she was place to seek solace of sexual and protective type. For Intuc she bore deeper values of philosophical nature and for Shrimant she was an object of sexual experiment to realize in vain his potency. The murder of Garbo by the end of the play is the upshot of the attempts on the part of the trio to regain the losing ground of control over the feminine world of pleasure represented by Garbo. They could not bear the thought that she killed the foetus. It was meant to offer a meaning to their lives in a specific way. She was already a part of the world they had created on the psychological level where they would never have the epiphany moments until this structure of the constructed world is disturbed by the violent act of Garbo. Intuc felt it could have been a real creation devoid of the false pretence on his part as he finds it in his poetry. He loses the only possibility of truly creative thing in its total originality. And thus also loses the only hope of being meaningful and useful in a philosophical manner. Shrimant and Pansy do not bear the loss of their fantasy. Shrimant especially loses the last opportunity to tell the world that he is father of the child and in this way he could maintain his position in the society that he is potent. It is Shrimant who stabs Garbo since he lost the hope against the problem for which Garbo was the only hope. The murder of Garbo takes place not on the account of the revenge that she killed a life and such acts are to be punished in a similar fashion. It is articulated mainly due to its immediate disturbance to the structure of patriarchal authority. Kate Millett in her book *Sexual Politics* making allusions from different cultures from China, Indian and Muslim countries talk about the male cruelties against women. She continues,

> The rationale which accompanies that imposition of male authority euphemistically referred to as "the battle of sexes" bears a certain resemblance to the formulas of nation at war, where any heinousness is justified on the grounds that the enemy is either an inferior species or really not human at all. The patriarchy mentality has concocted a whole series of rationales about women which accomplish this purpose tolerably well. And these traditional beliefs still invade our consciousness and affect our thinking to an extent few of us would be willing to admit (Millett 46).

It is very interesting to observe that the literature dealing with incest depicts such relationships with an aura of fear of destructive culmination. To name few, beginning with *Oedipus the Rex*, *Hamlet*, Gabriel Garcia Marquezs' *One Hundred Years of Solitude*, Raj Kamal Jha's *The Blue Bedspread* or Mahesh Dattani's *Thirty Days in September* have the relationship at the centre of thematic concern.

Oedipus is introduced mainly as a part of the elaboration on Freud's theory of Oedipus Complex. Hamlet's reluctance in thinking his mother to be an accomplice in the plot leading to death of his father poses the existence of conscious desire for one's mother whereas Oedipus' relation is not intentional and the realization results into tragic end. *One Hundred Years of Solitude* is the story of seven generation of the Buendia family.

Jose Arcadio Buendia and his wife Ursula who is cousin of Jose Arcadio, are aware of the possible vicious consequences of the incest relation they have engaged themselves in. Ursula tries to avoid the relations in vain. The myth, that such relationship yielded a child with a pig's tail and was eaten away by ants, haunts mind of the family. In the end of the narration of the trajectory a child is born out of incest relations with pig's tail and is eaten away by ants. The same destitute conditions of the partners engaged in the relationship can be seen in *The Blue Bedspread* and *Thirty Days in September*.

Of course, it is essential to recognize though the relationship is taboo, that the texts mentioned here from different cultures, pose different possibilities and discourses on the issue. Attempts can be made to put thread to pass through all the texts mentioned with the same theme with all their differences. Maya in *Thirty Days in September* is tormented by the memories of child abuse by her uncle who not only abused her but her mother too whereas Jha depicts a brother and sister with such relationship when the sister dies after giving birth to the child of his brother.

The common understanding, that the marriages among close relations are likely to result into having more possibilities of hereditary medical problems, is specifically considered today among many learned communities. But what incest is for a community is not incest for another community. The relationships considered as taboo in Hinduism, are not taboo in community like Muslim. Levi Strauss almost succeeded in telling in his book *The Raw and the Cooked* how incest is common in various cultures. It was an attempt to propose a poetics of the relationship forming a universal whole in vain. As we investigate the taboo, we understand that it has whole network and circle of reasons interconnected, which is of spacio-temporal nature. It is not easy to make an attempt like Strauss as we are aware of the diversity of conditions and situations in different places which have life governed by a specific set of values and principles.

It is not also so easy to catch them in their nudity in the age like this where time is rapidly changing and with it the values change gradually and more speedily in certain cases. The change in life style, city culture, industrialization, decentralization of joint family, the virtual reality generated by the media, the loss of traditional values creating a vacuum of desperation in the minds of people are few of the reasons that form the circle around which this investigation can move.

The end of Oedipus, though executed by himself and the suicide of Jocasta, the deaths caused due to procrastination by Hamlet, child being eaten away by ants in *One Hundred Years of Solitude* and traumatic conditions in which Maya lives even after many days of actual incidents of the abuse, are full of violence. Elkunchwar's play *Desire in the Rocks* meets with a tragic end where villagers beat Lalita and Hemkant brutally. Lalita sets the wooden mansion *(wada)* on fire where the couple dies.

The story of Hemkant and Lalita in *Desire in the Rocks* holds the significance of fundamental nature to Indian culture. It is the story of incest relationship between the brother Hemakant of thirty five and his sister Lalita of twenty in a general sense but issues like superstitions, human sacrifice, madness of Hemkant for the art of sculpture, childhood memories of Lalita, and violence are few of the issues the play deals with. Violence is sought as a solution to the fear of the possible bad effects of the incest. It becomes necessary to investigate how this culmination and its relation with the other factors that stimulate it or are affected by it, take place.

Probably one cannot maintain a standpoint by seeking a selection of an issue in its isolation denying the related 'circle of reason' for such an attempt is likely to result into fragmentation of investigation rather than bringing about the analysis of fruitful nature. It is exactly why, while investigating the violent incidents like human sacrifice, Lalita's decision about becoming a prostitute, villagers beating the beggar who agrees to bury their dead child, villagers's pelting stones and beating Hemkant and Lalita and Lalita's setting fire to the *wada* burning themselves dead, one has to concentrate on the specific issues which may not form a systematic whole or prove a help to complete a structural unity but offering a whole arena of network of diverse situations. Let's move on with this thinking to the close reading of the text that clearly offers the trinity of reasons which are related with society killing the human being indulging in incest relations, the human sacrifice due to superstitions and Lalita's exploitation, renunciation and the state of mind she arrives at.

In the play, the violent incidents are the end result of accumulation of intensity of certain feelings, beliefs and actions leading to the violation of certain social norms and values. The killing of the beggar along with her child and buried in the basement of the *wada* is purely the result of superstitions concerning the *vastushastra* and the various rituals like *vastushanti* exercises that have been performed since the time unknown. Many attempts of construction of the *wada* were made in vain and the necessity of human sacrifice was proposed. The beggar is captured with her child and both were buried in the basement of the *wada* and only after this sacrifice the construction reached its completion.

The incidents like human sacrifice can be frequently heard in today's time too. The question is what a set of thoughts gets into making of the blind belief that such sacrifice would gratify the evil spirits that (may) cause the trouble. The beginning of such ritual could be traced to the old traditions when human being gave and still giving animal sacrifice to please the natural forces and the specific gods. Human tendency towards violence in the case of communal riots appears to be very nature specific. Darwin explained how different animals developed from the same origin which was in accordance with natural selection. Requirements to be alive and to reproduce and struggle for existence brought changes in genes and the rate of the transformation increased with the intensity with which every generation struggled and craved for. However, this change according to Darwin does not thoroughly abandon the genes which were useful in a time long before though the same don't find any relevance in the present. This can also be related with the philosophical questions elaborated by Rousseau about human beings basically good and finding themselves in chains as they enter society and human beings being basically possessing bestiality which is moderated by social institutions. Golding showed how the children's bestiality turns uncontrollable in the absence of social control in his *Lord of the Flies*.

One more example could be cited here that of the couple of lion and lioness giving birth to a white cub in the jungle of Africa. The show on the channel Animal Planet about the cub does not concentrate on its strangeness. But rather comments on how it gets very difficult for the cub to hunt for his survival as he grows up. During the night, when the lions generally go for hunting taking the advantage of the darkness, the cub would be identified very easily in the darkness due to his white colour. The reasons behind such change which could not be called as mutations were stated that they were the genes of those ancestors who lived in the Ice Age where the white colour was an advantage for hunting the animals and that in turn assured the safety to their existence. In this way, the purpose of nature does not seem intelligible as to keep the genes existing through the broken chain of generation. It is not easy to call it a preparation on the part of Nature to have a tool ready for any possibilities. The question remains whether human beings have the traits of violence travelled from the time when man had to be violent for his/her existence, before the beginning of civilization which could also be called as socialization of violence.

In her article, "Kai Aahe Hinsachar?" Pratima Hawaldar offers the example of Chignon an anthropologist who studied Yanomamo community who lives in the southern part of Venezuela. "Chignon showed how violent life style of the community, the values imbibed through ages, develop a violent nature in the upcoming generation. He observed that more violent the person is, more he receives acceptance, prestige, and appreciation in the community. And the person intensifies his violence as to receive more respect in the community" (Hawaldar 01). He also showed how violent nature is developed through generation. It also becomes a part of their psyche.

The human sacrifice of the beggar could not just be said to be an act instigated by violent traits genetically present but such instincts generally function in accordance with the set of values and principles governing the social milieu, which is of spacio-temporal nature. In the play, people's beating to Hemkant and Lalita, are to be understood from the women mentioning about the incest relations by calling it 'filthy sin'. They are the embodiment of the social and religious forces which always look after the conformity. The incest relationship is considered a sin, a challenge to the set beliefs and religious values and teaching. Violence is always a preferred way to respond to such relations as violence is the act one chooses as one realizes that the logic, reason, meaningfulness and positive culmination from the argument is impossible. Of course, it is always an irrational tool. And above said preconditions consists of uniformity of thoughts justified by a philosophy which could appear flawless for those ones who inflict pain. The production of such a philosophy is culture-specific, community-specific, gender-specific and space-specific. The people in the village never approve the relation between the brother and sister. Besides it, the art of Hemakant that produced many statues in the form of nudity of Lalita are also disapproved. They destroy the statues. It is also a violent response by the society to the art which does not follow specific norms. The norms are so fortified that the change in time does not affect the values in certain cases. The example in Indian context can be clearly seen in caste system, religious values and places, concepts of morality, etc.

The character of Lalita undergoes a vital change. She almost becomes suicidal. She starts feeling that she has committed sin and she has to accept the evil effects of it. It is Hemkant who is responsible for the thinking of Lalita for she realizes that Hemkant does not love her but just makes use of her. She does not think her love for Hemkant a sin earlier. But when she realizes what she feels for him, he does not feel for her and he deliberately separates himself from her without getting involved in her since he thinks it is the way to understand something being objective. The realization of lack of love for her in Hemkant dawns on her. She does not tolerate her world of love conceived getting dismantled. Then her mind is full of thoughts of guilt, loss, the curse of the beggar, renunciation and self destruction as to get the punishment for the sin she has committed.

She thinks they both would have been dead, had Dadasaheb stayed in the *wada*. The existence of complex and phobic situations in which Lalita lives since her childhood, have prompted her to think it.

> Lalita: You're older than me. By fifteen years. That's why I feel scared. I've spent all these twenty years of my life just being scared.
>
> Hemkant: Were you afraid of Dadasahebz.
>
> Lalita: Petrified. After he died, I thought I was free of fear. But then the trustees and solicitors came. I was

afraid of them. I couldn't understand what they were
saying. Then you came, Hem. And I felt really free
(Elkunchwar 72).

She is afraid of the darkness through which Hemkant led
her to the *wada*. When she tells him how afraid she is of the
darkness and the ghostly appearance of the *wada*, Hemkant
not only ignores it but humiliates her for being so afraid of it.
He is much obsessed with the carvings, sculptures, designs on
the pillars, that he simply ignores frightened mind of Lalita
and describes the design on the stone and tells her how rich,
stately and prestigiously they appear. Lalita does not react to
this angrily. One can realize here that Hemkant can decipher
the degree of skills with which the stones or woods are carved
and can explain the grandeur in them but he fails to recognize
the mind of Lalita. He takes Lalita for granted to a state that for
Lalita too it appears to be natural. The situation is prerequisite
of a negative result. She says that she cannot take any decision
and she has lost the ability to take any decision since the time
she met him and tells him to all decisions about her. It is he
who brings Lalita to the village full of rocks and after listening
to reluctance of Lalita about staying there, he tells that the
village full of rocks, was beckoning him. It is challenge for the
artist like him. He says that he does not know about Lalita's
decision about staying there but he is going to stay there even
if Lalita does not accompany him.

The people of the village call them sinners. The violence
is mainly concerned here with the concept of sin. The concept
has its roots entangled in religious thinking. When Hemkant
tries to make it clear that Lalita is thinking that they have
sinned just because the dead child is born as it was the curse
for the every generation that dwelt in the mansion. He tries
to convince her that if the child would have been alive, she
would very fondly look after him and bring him up. It would

not have been a sin then. But she replies, "It's like a patch of leukoderma that has spread over the whole body. A few days of shame, but when the whole body is covered, what shame can there be? Sin once. Then it's over. That's not how it is. Sin never ends" (Elkunchwar 115)

Lalita thinks that by committing the sin, they have acted against the wish of Goddess and she says that the Goddess had come to her in her dream and "[t]hey want to punish us. The Goddess has commanded them to" (Elkunchwar 119).

For Lalita everything that is happening is a due course since they have sinned. When Hemkant tells her not to go out since the people are mad with rage. Lalita replies that is natural and the people are not to be blamed as they have broken all their conventions. It is noteworthy to find the same remarks by mother of Mala about the pain being unable to speak in Dattani's *Thirty Days in September* when she tells,

> "[F]or ten years! For ten years!! (*Pointing at the picture of God*). I looked at Him. I didn't feel anything, I didn't feel pained, I didn't feel pleasure. I lost myself to Him. He helped me…. By taking away all my feeling. No pain no pleasure, only silence…. But my fongue was cut off… I am dumb" (Dattani 55).

And the peak of her pain is felt when she jabs the sharp pieces of glass into her mouth making her mouth bleed. It is her punishment to herself for being unable to speak, being responsible for existing circumstances. Lalita tells the same to Hemkant.

> Lalita: Everything inside us is dead. It has smouldered within itself and burned down. To ashes. Ash is all that's left. A heap of ash. Not now. Never again (Elkunchwar 120).

Lalita picks up the torch and sets the mansion on fire. The couple dies. Lalita accepts it with no fear. Hemkant with his discovery of vanity of his idea of art, seems to admit his fault. Samik Bandyopadhyay in his introduction to Collected Plays of Mahesh Elkunchwar, attempts to bring a similar line of the violent act by Lalita and the people. He says,

> "The slow growth and eventual outburst of violence in/from the community matches the course of the pitched battle between Hem and Lalita, though maybe at a different level. Primeval passions lie at the root of both the passages of violence; the passion that holds a conventional society together against inroads from outside, and the passion that will hurl itself at the constraints to break free. It is the violent confrontation of the two passions that charges the Hem-Lalita relationship with a corrosive, self-destructive force" (Bandyopadhyay xvi-xvii).

However, the silence of the mob does not offer explicit elaboration on the violent action they do. But their violence can be thus explained by investigating the issues like superstitions, taboo, epiphany moments, mob psychology and the set of values and norms with which a society maintains its standards and violence is legitimated for the sustenance of those values and norms.

Holi has been already considered for the elements of revolt in the previous chapter. Revolt is a precondition of violent act. However every revolt does not end up in violence. The very use of the abusive language among the students in the play suggests violent possibilities of the issues that become the part of their discussions. The sheer disgust and anger against the authoritative regime of the principal who does not declare a holiday on the day of festival of *Holi*, leads through the amalgam of different subjective, political complexities, to the violent end with the suicide of a student after the torture he undergoes by the students on the campus. There are two incidents that prominently can be called as violent in the play. The first is the mental torture of the student named Anand by the students because he is the one who informs their names to the principal. The second incident is that of suicide by him.

Though violence by the students on the campus appears as the ultimate culmination of the pressure that is built up in them against the authoritarian power they could not directly challenge, it runs from subjective level to what Zizek calls it 'objective violence'. The two levels could be distinguished as the violence that appears to us in the form of personal aggression or Gopal slapping Anand on his face or Shrinivas bringing *sari* for Anand for making him wear it or Gopal threatening Anand saying that they will, "shave off his eyebrows. Tonsure his head. Tomorrow we'll drag him all over the campus in the sari! Go and tattle our names now! Go ahead!" (Elkunchwar 25)

Subjective form of violence is easily visible. It is the visibility of the form of various types of violence many a times deceives us making incomplete analyses of the basic nature of the violence that forms core of ideological framework of power. Power demands the others to be passive and expects to obey its orders with total submission. Any sort of denial to the power is handled with controlling measures. The principal does not expect any sort of opposition to the idea of having a guest lecture on the day of *Holi*. The protest against it is comes under the strict disciplinary action. On the other hand, the group of students engaged in the protest is the other. They are subject to the authoritative power of the management of the college. But they have their own structures of power within the group where power is exercised in the certain manner. They do not seem to believe and appreciate the subjugation of their 'right' to have the holiday. They indulge in violent act of making the

Holi fire. It is the very idea of resisting the suppression against which the students are protesting, becomes the tool when they express their anger against Anand. They torture him that leads to his suicide. In this way "violence inherits a system: not only the direct physical violence, but also the more subtle forms of coercions that sustain relation of domination and exploitation, including the threat of violence" (Zizek 10). The following remark of Ranjit reveals his violent ideas against the politicians and businessmen. He says, "I have just one effing ambition. Collect some potbellied ministers, some fat businessmen, and removing their clothes in some public square, kick them on their naked asses!" (Elkuchwar 13). Gopal says that there should be one correction in Ranjit's remark that after they are done with the kicking, rabid dogs should be set after them.

Zizek in his book emphasizes the need of understanding the real cause of violence. According to him out of the three forms of violence i.e. subjective, objective and symbolic, we tend to concentrate on the subjective form of violence caused by "the social agents, evil individuals, disciplined repressive apparatuses, fanatical crowds" (Zizek 10). He stresses the importance of understanding the objective nature of violence that exists in an isolated form. It seems to be alive independently. He thinks that the first form of visible violence occupies the larger space of common human mind since it is immediate to the vision and the impact of it is very vital. For Zizek, it is this form of violence, ultimately keeps us away from the proper analysis of the nature of ideological violence in the form of gender discrimination, racism, incitement, etc. It is why he advises "that one should resist the fascination of subjective violence… subjective violence is the just most visible of the three" (Zizek 11). It is in the same fashion if we consider the fact of homosexual tendencies grown between Shrivastav and Anand have become known to the other students on the campus and it is harboured antagonism towards the both especially towards the passive partner who is Anand. Kate Millett points out the peculiar violent characteristic of the sexuality. She says,

> But the taboo against homosexual behavior (at least among equals) is almost universally of far stronger force than the impulse and tends to effect a rechanneling of the libido into violence. This association of sexuality and violence is a particularly militaristic habit of mind. the negative and militaristic coloring of such men's house homosexuality as does exist, is of course by no means the whole character of homosexual sensibility (Millett 50).

It is this way in her larger argument regarding the strategies of patriarchal tradition that have been in a certain design always looked after sustaining its dominance over the female. It could be called in Zezekian term 'objective violence'. It is perhaps more true that one has to fight the objective form of violence rather than finding remedies for subjective one. Millett's disappointment is appropriate when she remarks about the course of even in *Doll's House* grows with the explicit implication of author's sexual orientations, traits of female character and 'masculine fixation':

> What is perhaps most discouraging of all is not even the masculine fixation on violence but the futility of the girls' sedentary dream, even its barrenness, for they sit awaiting the "intrusion of men and animals" and doing nothing at all – not even the "nurturance" expected of them (Millett 217).

In a broader perspective of observation of the criticism of dramatic and other writings in India and abroad a development of the stages of concentration could crudely be traced down to the subjective violence and objective violence as in the case of Millett mentioned above and the latest could be called as its symbolic state. Anshul Chandra in her essay "Vijay Tendulkar: A Critical Survey of his Dramatic World" the implications of violence that crosses the mere considerations of personal orientations which are specific to the situation at hand. She writes that Vijay Tendulkar's bifocal perspective on violence. According to her, *Gidhade,* has violence that tends to become 'an end in itself.' For her it is:

> the easiest way left for many ordinary citizens to cope up with their fractured selves and problems of living. No longer does violence come from ideology, faith or even self – interest. On the contrary, it seeks outlet in ideology, faith and perceived self – interest and latches on to these 'causes' to find public expression and legitimacy. In this paradoxical world, violence is prior to its causes (Quoted in Chakraborty 99).

In the chapter entitled "Fighting Bodies, Fighting Words: A Theory and Politics of Rape Prevention" from her book *Fighting Bodies, Fighting Words: A Theory and Politics of Rape Prevention,* Sharon Marcus's views recognize the objective violence but it does not rely on the mere recognition of the kind of violence but favours for counter action plan against the violence and refutes the views of Susan Brownmiller in her book *Against Our Will: Men, Women and Rape* that violence of rape exists in society as a 'fixed reality' and 'a fate worse than … death'. According to her, "Such view takes violence as a self – explanatory first cause and endows it with an invulnerable and terrifying facticity which stymies our ability to challenge and demystify rape… the apocalyptic tone which it adopts and the metaphysical status which it assigns to rape can only be feared or legally repaired, not fought" (Brownmiller 432).

The thesis of Zizek along with the various aspects mentioned above from different perspectives, leads us to reconsider the incidents of murder of Garbo in the play *Garbo*, the violence enacted by the crowd and suicidal end of Hemkant and Lalita in *Desire in the Rocks* and humiliation of Anand and suicide of Anand in *Holi*, the act of killing the tiger named *Sultan* by Rajshekhar and his suicide in the one act play *Sultan* and the murder of the old man in the play *Eka Mhataryacha Khun* by a woman and two men and the murder of Amrit in *Holi*.

On the superficial level these incidents appear to be the result of the immediate conflict that forms the background of the violent end. They are characterized with the issues like loss of potency in case of Shrimant who stabs Garbo, the mob's superstitious fear of evil befalling on their village due to the immoral act of taboo relation between the brother and sister, fear of restriction in the minds of student as Anand informs their names to the principal, Anand feeling too humiliated and unable to sustain self esteem against the act of the students making him wear a sari that attributes him the qualities of a woman, loss of meaning in life for Rajshekhar in *Sultan*, inability to get rid of the problems of life results in killing of the old man in *Eka Mhataryacha Khun* and the mystery that lies behind the release of Amrit and subsequent murder and possibility that the tribals will likely be accused for the murder of Amrit in *Holi*.

All the above mentioned situations in the plays do appear as a coherent part in the story line of the plays. They have their immediate cause of action. But all the incidents are the part of the larger structure of the network created by the system developed with the relationship among the producers and consumers in the society. As Zizek says the phenomenon of the 'objective violence' has undergone vital change with emergence of capitalism. However he feels the need of the idea of the violence to be thoroughly historicized. In Indian context, monarchy could be described as a controlling factor of means of production and thus ultimately the people in the disguise of kingship. In European context, kingship was successful in receiving the status next to God. In India they were favoured by Gods and they were said to possess the blessings of Gods and Goddesses. As the forms of governance went on changing in the course of time, the systems changed accordingly and with enlargement of the structure of society, population, emergence of new institutions, modernization, technology and so on.

With the industrial revolution in Europe, everything started changing very swiftly. Erick Hobsbawn in his *The Age of Revolution 1789 – 1848* talks how it affected the social structure and how there was the emergence of the two distinct classes of workers and capitalists. As Marx said how the superstructures are governed by the laws of the base and how superstructure itself is the very creation of the base. The base looks after the protection of its interest and creates the system in the form like that of judiciary and parliament that systematically protects the benefits of the base.

The interesting thing about the system is that it appears to be very natural and it is exactly the idea that prevents the individuals to look into its artificial nature and how it works with certain vested interests. Alex P. Schmid, in his book *Political Terrorism: A New Guide to Actors, Authors, Concepts, Data Bases, Theories, and Literature*, talks about definitive nature of terrorism and points out the variety of issues regarding violence and terrorism. He defines terrorism in a certain explanatory way. Accoridng to him it is anxiety-inspiring method of repeated violent action, employed by (semi-)clandestine individual, group, or state actors, for idiosyncratic, criminal, or political reasons, whereby—in contrast to assassination—the direct targets of violence are not the main targets. He rightly points out how randomly selected victims work as messengers. He continues:

Threat- and violence-based communication processes between terrorist (organization), (imperiled) victims, and main targets are used to manipulate the main target (audience(s)), turning it into a target of terror, a target of demands, or a target of attention, depending on whether intimidation, coercion, or propaganda is primarily sought (Schmid 28).

Amrit in *Party* is killed with a perfect plan. He had become the threat to the interests of the politicians. Amrit led a democratic way of opposing the intrusion into the rights of *adivasi*. Government was giving the land of *adivasi* to industry. It wanted to deforest the entire area. Many investors including the politicians like the chief minister himself were interested in the land. Amrit was a trouble to them and it was not easy for them to silence Amrit since he had a lawful way of protest but they managed to turn the silent protest into violent one and got Amrit arrested.

Naxalism is one of the issues that India is facing which could be called as the upshot of the political and economical imbalance since the time of British Raj. Naxalism is frequently characterized by its violent way of protest which perhaps is sought as an only means for solution to the problems of regional disparities and imbalances. Such situations bring the common people to the position of lookers on. They can do nothing but speak. Balram Halwai the protagonist in Arvind Adiga's novel *The White Tiger* apprehends the corrupt democracy and politics. He says it becomes no matter of wonder to see democracy and village people discussing the elections "like eunuchs discussing the *Kamasutra*" (Adiga 98).

Violence becomes an only way out for the section of society trapped under the fortified system of power. The two forms of violence one enacted as a form of resistance to the authoritative regime and sought as an only way out whereas the second is the state's organized violence in the form of ideology. Amrit became the victim of state's violence whereas the Naxalism undertook the violent way and began to attack the base of the superstructure. Of course one must never forget that it is the last weapon one has to choose realizing well the possible threat to one's existence. An authoritative People's Daily article, poetically captioned "Spring Thunder Over India", hailed Naxalbari and laid down the line for the Indian People's war against the four "big mountains" – imperialism, Soviet re-visionism. Feudalism and bureaucrat-capitalism.

The changing nature of economy has brought but more disheartening and challenging conditions making their lives impossible and state's totalitarian regime poses political impossibility. In his article *in Economical and Political Weekly* in August 1972 Mohan Ram emphasized, "[W]ith the arrest of Charu Muzumdar, just as five years ago they gleefully pronounced revolution in India dead with failure of the Naxalbari up-rising, as though Naxalbari was the beginning and end of the Indian revolution. It was neither; at best it could be vested with a certain symbolism" (Ram 1471).

On the other hand, holding on factual line of recent development in Naxal crises in November 2008 PCAPA (People's Committee Against Police Atrocities) led mass protest against police brutality. The spokespersons of PCAPA Asit Mahato declared the outfit would no longer continue democratic protest. "After continuous torture by the joint forces, the PCAPA has decided to combat the forces" (Mittal 30).

However the depth of the fear imbedded in such statements provides us with the revolutionary potentials that exist in the country. Indian mindset requires breaking through the shackles of human civilization oscillates between the 'Freedom from Fear' and the 'Fear of Freedom'. "The spirit of man ... is free but contextuality of freedom is always restraining factor in the operation of freedom. If freedom means the birth-right to an individual to act without inhabitations of control, the free will to act operates in given context. The contest may be physical, existential, political and social. Freedom without context is too abstract to contemplate" (Mohanty 220).

Shrimant and Anand's articulation of violence is a part of the similar structure of gender. They have had the masculine conceptions descending from the thought line of patriarchal tradition that unconsciously and invisibly imposes certain responsibilities on them. It is how every 'man' gets entangled into them and so the 'woman'. Their actions of violence do get the motivations from the thinking of sustenance of the power being male and it is the condition that made them think themselves powerful as far as potency, honour, meaningfulness and self esteem in society and personal life is concerned. They cannot manage the threat to these illusions and delusions which are the product of the larger structure of ideology with non violence. Violence becomes legitimate tool for them to react with and it is how Shrimant can make use of violence because being a man he qualifies himself to make use of it and Anand on the other hand cannot tolerate the loss of it and is able to take another decision of killing himself. For Anand the shameful situation he lived becomes a stigma he cannot live with in society. It so happens not only on the pure level of rational thinking but also on the level the way one fantasizes the world around oneself. Theses fantasies which change from person to person with no regular method very basically provide human beings with prerequisites for the possible reaction appropriated by the stimuli from immediate course of time. The fantasies realize the desire in a systematic form and looks after fulfilling them and so to say more elaborately

> "rather, its function is similar to that of Kantian 'transcendental schematism': a fantasy constitutes our

> desire, provides its co-ordinates; that is, it literally
> 'teaches us how to desire'... fantasy meditates between
> the formal symbolic structure and the positivity of
> the objects we encounter in reality – that is to say,
> it provides a 'schema' according to which certain
> positive objects in reality can function as objects of
> desire, filling in the empty places opened up by the
> formal symbolic structure" (Zizek 7).

It appears true when it is seen how human mind intends to seek violence as a tool to fight against any possible danger to the 'schema'. It of course also depends on what positions one holds in society, what gender the person belongs to, what category in regard to religion, caste, creed, race one represents. For Anand and Lalita's becomes an action of resistance when the formal order of realizing desire gets disturbed while for Shrimant it becomes counter action with involvement of violence.

Exhibition of sexuality has been one of the ways of the indicators of the repulsive tendencies. The use of sexually abusive language is not aimed at only attacking the other person but it aims at achieving certain desired effects. It challenges the sexual potency of a person, which in a complex way is ambiguous and full of uncertain of its meaning and nature. However there exists a lifelong confusion and doubt about the sexual capability and strength in one's mind especially before one gets acquainted with sexual experience. It is here the sexual fantasies play an important role. It has been the result of sum of the culturally constructed ideas of sexuality i.e. manliness or feminine.

There is one more aspect to the violence in the form of suicide committed by Lalu in *Holi*. It mainly connects with his sexual orientation. Jonathan Gardiner, in his essay on "Why are homosexuals committing suicide" writes that the suicide problem in the homosexual community is not because that common people think such behavior as odd or unnatural. Sometimes it is even thought as sinful. He proposes that homosexuals like Anand commits suicide

> when they are discovered or mocked at because they know the behavior to match the behavior is wrong, and have no self-control to correct their behavior to match what they believe to be right. In the end, when people point this out through ridicule, they are incapable of dealing with the cognitive dissonance and are led to believe that only suicide can help them escape the anguish of that state of mind" (Quoted in Kulkarni 223).

This opinion of Jonathan holds truth at a greater level about the crucial problems of homosexual community. It is not the only culmination. However, they also develop certain psychological tendencies which are not considered normal.

The above discussion brings about the idea of third division of kind of violence and thus the analyses of violence moves ahead of the subjective and objective form of violence. It becomes necessary to investigate the role of other agencies regarding the articulation of violence. It has always been stated and is presented to us as the beginning of civilization was also the beginning of humanism that brought the difference between human beings and animals. Violence was one of the issues that have been brought to the line of comparison by the philosophers like Descartes. It is the mainstream tradition of thinking that the one of the greatest invention of human mind i.e. language or the symbolic order has always been working as the medium to offer solution to the barbarity of human mind; it brings the order and systematization to irrational behavior. And more basically it is the order of recognition and meaning that helps human understand the world in a certain way.

The role of language is significant in shaping the way we perceive the world and the reality of the world. In fact it is the language itself which is the medium through which every understanding is created and activated. Without the language we simply cease to exist on a certain levels. The language is not self sufficient. It could be called as the mistake on the part of the thinkers who conceived language as "the medium of reconciliation and mediation of peaceful co-existence... In language, instead of exerting direct violence on each other, we are meant to debate, to exchange words, and such and exchange, even when its aggressive, presupposes a minimum recognition of the other" (Zizek 1). While making references to Jean-Marie Muller, Zizek mentions the two ways how renunciation of violence is sought as speaking is the foundation and structure of socialization that happens due to the renunciation of violence and even if it happens it happens due to a radical perversion of humanity when "language gets infected by violence and it happens under the influence of contingent 'pathological' circumstances which distort the inherent logic of symbolic communication" (Zizek 2).

The close reading of the episode wherein the violent action is performed, suggests the certain kind of failure in human reconciliation. Taking into consideration the whole discourse of subjective and objective violence, one could also find how the symbolic order also has its share in bringing about the violence in the form of murder that Shrimant commits and suicide committed by Anand and Lalita.

Walter Benjamin wrote "Critique of Violence" raising the question whether any non-violent resolution of conflict is possible. His answer is to the question is positive and he writes, "there is a sphere of human agreement that is non-violent to the extent that it is wholly inaccessible to violence: the proper sphere of 'understanding', language" (Quoted in Zizek 1). Language in mainstream thought line, is considered a true resolution for the problem of violence and it has been the accepted idea of function of language that is taken as one of the advantages and characteristics of civilization.

It will not be thus difficult for one to recognize on the superficial level the authenticity of application of the idea to the conflicts in the plays as discussed so far. It is the lack of proper sphere of communication through language that could be said to be a major problem in avoiding the violent way out for the non adjustable situations. Before Shrimant stabs Garbo, it has become impossible for Garbo to get along with the logic of her life with the lack of availability of linguistic resolution which she puts it, "I will not be happy with anybody now... too late for that...mind has grown too calculating...If ever I feel momentary tenderness for anybody, ... You know what suffering will follow" (Elkunchwar 57).

What happens at the time of murder of Garbo by Shrimant is to be seen in a certain form where Shrimant loses access to any meaningful culmination of understanding of the situation he gets caught in. When he tells Garbo that he was going to look after her child, she makes it clear that if it would have been done, it would not be out of compassion but only as cover for his lost manhood. It is here Shrimant's conflict grown within him is fortified. When he does not find the proper recognition to his intention by Garbo, he flares at her abusive defense and it is the immediate position he could adopt. He says to her, "A whore. That's what you are. A whore... I'll fling a few paise at you and make you dance naked for me (Elkunchwar 63).

Before the moment of murder comes, Shrimant once again tells her to come to him and he would take care of her. It was a constant attempt from Shrimant to seek a meaning to the life he is living. To him to be able to tell the world that he is a father of a child, would mean a meaning to hold on to a position in society. It means his establishment in society as a potent male. The death of the child makes him lose the only opportunity and it angers him. His vain attempts to go to prostitute and failure in sexual satisfaction have already put him in frustrated mindset. It is also one of the reasons in which he loses the resolution. It is however also a culture specific creation of notion of masculinity and potency. Being impotent leaves a human being in a restless state of mind and is always connected with death. No alternative is offered in this regard.

Now it is interesting to observe that it is not a straight way out to seek a violent response against certain impossibility of positivity of action. One does utilizes various means before the violent culmination of the course of action. In a social condition, it is not always impossible to seek for a situation that could be called as safe. There are many techniques and methods which are deployed to bring oneself in an advantageous position. They are sought with selection of lying, denial, belief, pretence, hope, procrastination, patience, honesty, reason and 'willing suspension of disbelief' and so on. Shrimant stabs Garbo only when she finishes off the last chance of him possessing her in order to bring a meaningful order to his life and starts going out of the house.

In case of Lalita in *Desire in the Rocks,* it may not be a different experience. When we realize it is the same state of mind where Lalita reaches giving up for the impossibility of any positive resolution of situation, and says, "Everything inside us is dead. It has smouldered within itself and burned down... Not now. Never again (Elkunchar 120). It is Lalita in the play who puts the *wada* on fire thus seeking a violent death of both of them. Before she comes to the terms with suicidal state of mind, she suffers from a series of events in which all the epitomes of her belief get dismantled. Loss of mother and dominating father begin the trouble for Lalita from early childhood. After the death of father, she could not come out of the trauma she always suffered from. Her brother Hemkant was the only solace to her and she found a meaningful existence with him. She is ready to go with him to such a village where there is nothing that comforts her on any level. It only with the thought she has Hemkant whom she has offered her body and mind whole heartedly.

The events that follow her realization of Hemkant's mind that he has messed up the idea of art with life and given away the dead child to the beggar to bury it; she jabs the sharp pieces of glass into her mouth making her mouth bleed; she becomes a whore and allow people to misuse her body and puts the mansion on fire. Her statement about the impossibility of resolution becomes very clear, "It's like a patch of leukoderma that has spread over the whole body. A few days of shame, but when the whole body is covered, what shame can there be? Sin once. Then it's over. That's not how it is. Sin never ends" (Elkunchwar 115). What she means from 'sin never ends' is unavailability of any logical, meaningful resolution to her problem of unholy love she has with her brother.

It is essential here to recognize as long as she knew and believed in the idea that if it is the true love between the two, it does not matter what social structure of relation they belong to. Lalita's was the psyche that already sought shelter under immediate object of desire that helped her to forget the tormenting memory of past she lived. Her brother was for her the only person she trusted and knew. It had already appropriated the illegitimacy of incest relationship. However it could last only till the destruction of the belief.

Lalita's religious belief of self punishment would be the only way out to repent the sin prove key in her directions of actions. These occupy her mind and when it also does not satisfy her completely, she comes to a certain state of mind where impossibility of linguistic resolution becomes reality. The same is the case with the violence that takes place in the plays like *Holi* and *Party* on a level where a mob of students is involved in the first case and in the other it is system that triggers the death of Amrit. In both the situations the impossibility of communicative resolution is null.

Though this mainstream thought line seems to be firmly logical, there are certain standpoints from which it is not always very difficult to recognize the language plays in our life on various levels right from the bringing about the concept of reality to the making it realize in itself and doubt about it (if at all one can) in language itself. Zizek continues it saying,

> When we perceive something as an act of violence, we measure it by a presupposed standard of what the "normal" non – violent situation is – and the highest form of violence is the imposition of this standard with reference to which some events appear as "violent". This why language -itself, the very medium of non – violence, of mutual recognition, involves unconditional violence (Zizek 2).

Zizek summarizes the standpoints regarding the relation between language and violence, assumed by the philosophers like Fredrick Jameson, Freud, Lacan, Heidegger, Plato, Wittgenstein, Kierkegaard and Nietzsche and so on. It however comes to an unresolved understanding of problematic of plurality of views on the issue. He notes how Lacan at times has to borrow and rely on certain ideas of thinkers like Kierkegaard or Heidegger in order to bring about a balanced discourse on the 'truth' of role of language in violence. The crux of the conflict regarding the role and responsibility of language in violence relies on the idea of violence that exits in language and violence as a biological reality. Zizek in this regard states the views of Lacan that,

[i]n a human being, desires lose their mooring in biology, they are operative only insofar as they are inscribed within the horizon of Being sustained by language; however, in order for this transposition from the immediate biological reality of the body to the symbolic space to take place, it has to live a mark of torture in the body in the guise of its mutilation (Zizek 5).

As the conflict is harbored between the symbolic and the real, Lacan and Heidegger have different views on the nature and role of *jouissance* and its relation with being. Realizing the complexity of the issue and the difference between the "two deaths" Lacan has to come to the terms with challenging philosophy itself with due recognition saying *jouissance* as something which, "although it is far from being simply external to language, resists symbolization, remains a foreign kernel within it, appears within it as a rupture, cut, gap, inconsistency or impossibility" (Zizek 7). Like the issue of desire and sexuality, the issue of violence is crucial in the plays of Elkunchwar. These issues always bear plural nature of significance. Purnima Kulkarni looks at the play in different view as she says that subalterns speaks in the play. Accoridng to her, Elkunchwar's, "like Brecht, purpose of drama is to teach us how to survive by familiarizing them with the social problems and simultaneously distancing them from the emotions of the characters" (Kulkarni 223). The didactic part of this statement could be doubted but the skills and certain influences Elkunchwar succeeds in offering through his dramatic world are of high value.

Works Cited

Adiga, Arvind. *The White Tiger.* New Delhi: Harper Collins, 2008. Print.

Ambedkar, B. R. "Mr. Russell and the Reconstruction of Society." Rev. of *Principles of Social Reconstruction.* Journal of the Indian Economic Society 01. July, 1918: 16. Print.

Bandyopadhyay, Samik. Introduction. *Collected Plays of Mahesh Elkunchwar Vol. I,* By Elkunchwar. New Delhi: 2009. Print.

Brownmiller, Susan. *Against Our Will: Men, Women and Rape.* New York: Fawcett Columbine, 1975. Print.

Chakroborty, Kaustav, ed. *Indian Drama in English.* New Delhi: PHI Learning Pvt. Ltd., 2011. Print.

Cusack, Catherine. *Theatre and Violence.* London: Palgrave Mcmillan, 2013. Print.

Dattani, Mahesh. *Collected Plays. Vol. II.* New Delhi: Penguin Books India, 2005. Print.

Elkunchwar, Mahesh. *Collected Plays of Mahesh Elkunchwar Vol. I.* New Delhi: Oxford University Press, 2009. Print.

..,. *Collected Plays of Mahesh Elkunchwar Vol. II.* New Delhi: Oxford University Press, 2011. Print.

Hobsbawm, Eric. *The Age of Revolution 1789 – 1848*. New York: Vintage Books. 1996. Print.

Fanon, Franz. *The Wretched of the Earth*. Harmondsworth: Penguin Books, 1965. Print.

Foucault, Michel. *Discipline and Punish: The Birth of Prison*. Trans. Alen Sheridan, London: Penguin Books, 1977. Print.

..., *The History of Sexuality. Vol. I*. New York: Vintage Books. 1990. Print.

Hawaldar, Pratima, "Kai Aahe Hinsachar?" *Hinsa Te Dahashatwad*. ed. Kunte, Pune: Diamond Publications, 2009. Print.

Hobsbawm, Eric. *The Age of Revolution 1789 – 1848,* New York: Vintage Books. 1996. Print.

Jha, Raj Kamal. *The Blue Bedspread*. London: Picador. 1999. Print.

Kulkarni, Purnima. "Subalterns Speak in Mahesh Elkunchwar's *Holi*". *Contemporary Discourse* 6:1 (2015): 219. Web. 20 Oct, 2015.

Machiavelli. *The Prince*. Trans. C. E. Detmold. Kent:1997. Print.

Marcus, Sharon. *Fighting Bodies, Fighting Words: A Theory and Politics of Rape Prevention,* Columbia: Routledge. 2002. Print.

Millette, Kate. *Sexual Politics*. Urbana and Chicago: University of Illinois Press, 1970. Print.

Mittal, Tusha. "How a Deaf Ear is Turning Plughshares to Swords". *Tehelka* 44 (2009): 30. Print.

Mohanty, Prafull. K. "Freedom as Identity: The Literature of Rising". *Indian Literature, Sahitya Akademi's Bi-Monthly Journal* 1. (2009): 220. Print.

"On the Principles of Political Violence and Anti-Fascist Action" Diss. University of Manchester, Web. 19 July, 2015.

Ram, Mohan, "Five Years After Naxalbari." *Economic and Political Weekly 7* Web (1972): 1471.

Sartre, Jean-Paul. Preface. *The Wretched of the Earth.* by Franz Fanon. Harmondsworth: Penguin Books: (1965): 23-26. Print.

Schmid, A. P. and Jongman A. J. *Political Terrorism: A New Guide to Actors, Authors, Concepts, Data Bases, Theories, and Literature. New Brunswick: Transaction Books.2005.* Print.

Strauss, Levi. *The Raw and the Cooked.* Trans. John and Doreen Weightman. Plon. 1964. Print.

"Violence." Def. 2b. *Oxford Advanced Learner's Dictionary.* 8th ed.(2010). 1719. Print.

Zizek, Slovej. "Language, Violence and Nonviolence." *International Journal of Zizek Studies* 2:3 (2008): 01. Web. 21 Jan, 2014.

..,. *Violence.* New York: Picador, 2008. Print.

Chapter **V**
CONCLUSION

T his research work consists of the analysis of the issues, forces and various cultural factors that form the core of social and individual behavior namely sexuality and aggressive responses in the form of revolt and violence. From the collections of more than a dozen plays written by Mahesh Elkunchwar and collectively published by Oxford University Press were mainly considered for the analysis. They were selected as per their thematic concerns and analyzed under each subsequent chapters i.e. desire, revolt and violence. However, the plays like *Yatanaghar* which are not translated are also considered for certain references and thematic concerns.

In the beginning of the present research work, certain observations are registered that suggest the tendency of research and critical views regarding the study of Indian drama in general. The survey and history of critical thoughts about Indian drama writing, has been recognized for having certain peculiarities like that of random selection of writers writing purely in English and selective dramatists like Tendulkar and Karnad which are translated in English. There have been limitations in the contemporary critical writings as far as the history of drama writing in India is concerned. The limitations mainly are about inclusive writing and rewriting of critical history of Indian drama in English and translation.

Text, context, author and reader are locus of all literary and critical theories. They formed the basis of importance in certain approaches. The whole critical thought about literary analyses could be divided among the four. The singularity of a thought or a locus is always questionable. The nature or the genre in which the text is formulated presents different possibilities of perceptions, meaning, effects and 'uncertainty' in meaning. Elkunchwar has been controversial when he declares that the play belongs to the actors that perform it. This view is predominated by the personal experience of the dramatist and it is largely related with the performance of the play in theatre. The strength, nature, style and techniques of dialogue delivery of the actors are observed having more effect on the text and meaning implied by the author. However, Elkunchwar's thought of assigning the significance excludes the importance of other crucial factors that form the core of the performance, creation of the text and generation of overall meaning.

Elkunchwar becomes an important playwright in Marathi play writings among Khanolkar, Tendulkar, Shirvadkar, Gadkari, Kanitkar, Alekar and others. Among the playwrights, Tendulkar, Alekar and Elkunchwar are considered significant as far as professional theatre and modernism in Indian drama are concerned. The research work has also acknowledged the significant contribution of other dramatic traditions and their under currents which are non Brahminical. Among such traditions, *Dalit* theatre is the most prominent. Its prominence is of higher nature that forms the centre and beginning of overall *dalit* writings and movements in India.

A chronological survey of writings of Elkunchwar has been sought that includes inclusive study of his plays beginning with his one act play *Sultan*. Elkunchwar emerges as a philosopher and a messenger who attempts to present the core of Indian values and its rich tradition. He presents the ethos, in all its variety, challenges of meaning of life and gratification of senses and ultimate satisfaction. He seems to be largely affected by the idea of creation in its various forms. The idea of creation in the form of writing, arts like sculpting, reproduction have formed the basis of most of his plays like *Garbo, Desire in the Rocks, Autobiography, Party, Zumbar*, etc. He deals with the most significant part in the process of creation i.e. the value of the creation, the nature of its stimuli, art for life sake, art for art and significance and relationship between human life and art.

In addition to it, 'death' has been a major issue in the writings of Elkunchwar. There are deaths and suicides in many of his plays. The events of death in various forms bring about formative sense in readers' and audience's mind. In this regard, Elkunchwar seems to be attracted toward the absurdist theatre and its implications towards life. The deaths in his plays are not driven by simple and direct effects of events. They are rather of absurd nature and also a result of psychological and philosophical conflicts in human mind. Most of the times, the conflicts are related with idea of creation in different forms, the idea of ultimate satisfaction, the idea of love and the idea of happiness.

Elkunchwar's success on professional theatre and as a matured playwright largely rests on the questions he raises through the conflicts faced by his characters. The evasive nature of religions, human relationships and meaning of life largely affected by external factors like technological changes and degradation of traditional ways of life are today's most crucial issues that receive voice in Elkunchwar's plays. The change in time and culture brings with the vivid realization of certain psychological and philosophical conflicts in human mind. Elkunchwar's presentation of the issues becomes more effective and authentic when he shows that the characters that face such conflicts have realized the uncertainty of meaning of happiness and satisfaction and meaning of overall life in general. The stimuli for the production of such feelings in the minds of the characters is instigated by the realization received externally about the lack of uniformity of thoughts that otherwise holds together human mind with certain meaning, certain ideas of happiness embedded in family ties, religious beliefs, positivity of social institutions and strength of human relationships. For Lalita, it is her brother Hemkant who brings the idea of this type of detachment and fragmentation of uniformity of the beliefs. Same is the case with Chandrashekhar, Anand and others who meets the destructive end.

Elkunchwar's choice of 'desire', 'revolt' and 'violence' as thematic traits in his plays has valid bases of human tendencies. The culmination of human life, as identified by the author, is never devoid of these issues. It is seen and analyzed that the sexuality of general and taboo kind, revolt in its multiple implications and nature and violence in the forms of suicide and murders as shown in Elkunchwar's plays, have cultural, psychological, political, social and discursive orientations that function in a way that brings about certain responses.

Desire and sexuality form a stronger core in human life. The evolution of idea of sexuality along with the growth of civilization has not been a process of logical rendering. Certain cultural aspects like silences and secrecy were observed due to various reasons. In strong religious senses, desires and sexuality were considered obscene and forbidden. These were the important stages in the history of civilization as far as the issue of desire and its satisfaction is concerned. The text like

Kamasutra by Vatsyayana gives the idea of certain time when ideas of desire and sexuality were allowed to be documented. But time changed and so did the common perception of the issue change. In European context, Foucault observes how certain tendencies probed in and how Victorian regime carefully confined sexuality and never allowed bodies to have 'display of themselves'. It lost the certain frankness about sexuality.

It is not only through the selection of issues like incest relationship between Hemkant and Lalita in *Desire in the Rocks*, Baby and her brother Ramesh in *Yatanaghar*, homosexual desires in *Holi* and *Garbo* where desire of the objects are Anand and Pansy and explicit treatment of sexuality in the plays like *Garbo, Reflection, As One Discardeth Clothes...*, *Party, Rudravarsha* and *Ek Osad Gaon*, Elkunchwar tries to present a picture of Indian society in particular and human life experience in general but the characters like Intuc and Lalita become the voice of the playwright and it is through their opinions and dialogues certain aura of sense and understanding of author's mind could be fathomed.

In the play *Garbo*, while insisting on letting Garbo to be what she is, Intuc emphasizes that they should first know what they themselves really are. According to him, this would be a 'sound enough basis for their relationships with her'. The following is the remark by Intuc that could be called as an underlined thought as far as discourse on sexual desires is concerned. According to Intuc all the business about woman being an enigma and all that is a myth. He calls it a bit of literary truth. He contributes to man-woman relationship saying once one understands a woman; one does not want to look at her again. He adds that once one explores her, the thrill is gone. Here 'explore' has significance of 'sex'. Intuc's philosophy about women takes an ultimate turn when he comments rather gender biased remark that a woman should be able to satisfy you fully, and yet withhold a part of her from you.

It becomes both inner voice of the playwright and his effective way of registering his observations through the characters. The same could be found in the play *Desire in the Rocks* when Lalita realizes the void in the nature of their relationship and says the experience she lived was like a 'patch of leukoderma'. It has spread over the whole body. She tells that it is a matter of a few days of shame but when the whole body is covered, there remains no shame. It becomes whole of you. It is a sin once and its event is over but it remains as long as one lives. It does not get over.

For the evaluation of the issues of desire and sexuality, his plays like *Garbo, Holi, As One Discardeth Clothes…, Desire in the Rocks, Flower of Blood* and *Autobiography* are analyzed. There have been various objects of desire in the plays. As mentioned earlier, the relations also include relationships like incest and homosexuality. For almost all the characters, the beginning of the conflict is instigated due to the problems with the object of desire, loss of object of desire, confusion in deciding the object of desire, conflict between the couple and the conflict in their object of desire and lastly it is the loss of desire itself.

It is referred to Zizek's ideas about the role of fantasies in construction and realization of desires in human life. He writes in his book *The Plague of Fantasies* referring to Kantian 'transcendental schematism' that a fantasy constitutes our desire, provides its co-ordinates and also teaches us how to desire. He explains the role of fantasy and how it meditates between the formal symbolic structure and the positivity of the objects we encounter in reality. According to him, fantasy provides a 'schema' according to which certain positive objects in reality can function as objects of desire, filling in the empty places opened up by the formal symbolic structure.

It is applicable to sexualities like incest, homosexuality and prostitution.

There are myriad forces that function in ways which can never satisfactorily be adjusted to our predetermined categories like logic and reasoning. It is also recognized that such forces are not entirely independent. They are limited in particular structure which could exist in a certain way at a certain period of time. For example, dramatists like Shirvadkar, Khanolkar, Tendulkar and Elkunchwar have a type of literary production in a form of dramatic writing that does not limit itself limited arena of social structure they are part of nor is there always a constant effort for making their writings politically correct and intentionally fortified or manufactured.

Elkunchwar artistically deals with the realism which is both visible and invisible in the structures of various relationships. In a general sense, this act by any author becomes a particular form of a 'gesture' that does not necessarily go with the common perception of reality. Such gestures are always probing and encroaching the established 'ways of seeing'. It could be called as a revolt in a certain sense. With this understanding, it becomes necessary to realize that the use of word revolt is manifold and as far as this research work is concerned, it is used in both the ways i.e. revolt in general sense and revolt in literary sense which could be written as 'literary revolt'. What difference does matter between the two is that of origin and inspiration of the revolt.

Elkunchwar banged on the scene of Marathi play writing with a kind of bold plays like *Garbo, Desire in the Rocks, As One Discardeth Old Clothes…, Yatanghar* and *Holi.* The act of dealing issues of incest, homosexuality and desires exhibiting sexual cravings as exta-marital affairs was an act of revolt on the part of the dramatist. It was rather a very conscious effort by the playwright as far as the play Garbo is concerned.

However, the plays like *Garbo, Holi, Sultan, As One Discardeth Old Clothes…, Autobiography, Party* and *Desire in the Rocks* are considered for the analyses of theme of revolt. Lalita, Garbo, Aai and Vasanti are female characters that bring about the revolt which is of dual type. They act against the forces created by the society and the individuals around them. However, the second type of revolt becomes inevitable as the female characters realize their subjugation mainly caused by patriarchal and male dominated society. Few references are made for feministic interpretations of the texts to Kate Millett's book *Sexual Politics*. The forces stimulate the female characters' identity crises, notions of revenge, renunciation and eventually a revolt.

The visibility of violence is noticeable in Elkunchwar's plays. Many a times, Elkunchwar ends his plays with devastated and confused state of mind of his characters culminating in destruction. The destruction takes place in the form of suicide and murder. The events of suicide form the core of the play like *Sultan, Desire in the Rocks* and *Holi.* However, the web of reasons and forces that stimulate such self destruction is of varied nature.

The act of suicide is mainly an act of violence. The only difference that lies in the act is that the object of the pain to be inflicted on is not someone else; it is rather oneself. It could also be justified in terms of Indian legal system.

History plays a vital role in the deciding the nature of aggressive and violent responses in a nation at a larger level. Colonialism and imperialism left a deep impact on minds of the colonized. The process of freedom was never devoid of violence. Process of decolonization involved violence and its legitimacy in different forms. In *The Wretched of the Earth*, Franz Fanon talks about such legitimacy. In the country like India, there have been myriad episodes in its history that saw much bloodshed. Recent history in relation with the participation too involved too much killing and massacre. The intensity of these memories is still felt through literature and movies. Post colonial conditions can never be judged and analyzed without paying due considerations to the process of colonization and decolonization.

However the issue of violence in the selected play is considered with multiple views. In *Garbo*, there are two events in which violence takes place i.e. killing of the fetus by Garbo and at the end of the play murder of Garbo by Shrimant. The first form of violence is a subjective violence enacted by Garbo. The subjective violence however is predominated by objective violence in the form of social and economic structures.

In *Desire in the Rocks*, violence is sought as a solution to the fear of the possible side effects of the incest. It becomes necessary to investigate how this culmination and its relation with the other factors that stimulate it or are affected by it, take place. Lalita before setting the mansion of fire, allows much violence on her body. External violent forces are also visible in the play. However, it is internal conflict of Lalita that instigates ultimate end to their lives.

Though violence by the students on the campus in *Holi* appears as the ultimate culmination of the pressure that is built up in them against the authoritarian power they could not directly challenge, it runs from subjective level to what Zizek calls it 'objective violence'. The two levels could be distinguished as the violence that appears to us in the form of personal aggression or Gopal slapping Anand on his face or Shrinivas bringing *sari* for Anand for making him wear it or Gopal threatening Anand saying that they will shave off his head and eyebrows and dragging him all over the campus in the sari. The objective violence further could be explained in words of Jonathan Gardiner who talks about why homosexuals are committing suicides. For Jonathan the main reason behind homosexuals' suicides is lack of 'self control to correct their behavior' and incapability of dealing with 'cognitive dissonance'.

As far as the murder of Amrit in *Party* is concerned, it is also the objective violence that makes the murder happen. It is an obvious and vivid act of political violence. It is also observed how language itself is a strong tool in exercising violence. The structure of language, its meaning production and functions consist of a large degree of imbalance. It is true when Zizek writes in his article "Language, Violence and Nonviolence" that the language which is called medium of nonviolent reconciliation and proper sphere of understanding and mutual recognition involves unconditional violence. This view proves very helpful not only to analyze the issue of violence but also other conflicts that form the base of many plays of Elkunchwar.

Elkunchwar plays due to their rich content and subject matter will remain truly great literary work of art. They could be studied with variety of approaches and will still remain a challenge to the critics as they have at their core the most delicate and incomprehensive issues about human world of emotions and experiences.

A Select Bibliography

Primary Sources:

Elkunchwar, Mahesh. *Collected Plays of Mahesh Elkunchwar Vol. I.* New Delhi: Oxford University Press, 2009. Print.

Elkunchwar, Mahesh. *Collected Plays of Mahesh Elkunchwar Vol. II.* New Delhi: Oxford University Press, 2011. Print.

Elkunchwar, Mahesh. *Maunrag.* Mumbai: Mauj Prakashan, 2005. Print.

Elkunchwar, Mahesh. *Paschimprabha.* Aurangabad: Chakshu Prakashan, 2006. Print.

Elkunchwar, Mahesh. *Sanwadacha Suwawo: Conversation with Principal Ram Shewalkar.* Pune: Rajhans Prakashan, 2009. Print.

Elkunchwar, Mahesh. *Two Plays: Reflection, Flower of Blood.* Calcutta: Seagull Books, 1989. Print.

Secondary Sources:

Books:

Adiga, Arvind. *The White Tiger.* New Delhi: Harper Collins, 2008. Print.

Amrite, Sandhya. *Elkunchwarachi Natyasrushti.* Napur: Vijay Prakashan, 1995. Print.

Aristotle. *Nicomachean Ethics.* New York: Dover Publications, Inc., 1998. Print.

Artaud, Antonin. *The Theatre and Its Double.* Trans. Victor Corti, Richmond: Alma Clasics, 2010. Print.

Arvikar, Sanjay. *Shodh Elkunchwaranchya Kalakruticha.* Pune: Padmagandha Prakashan, 2001. Print.

Baldwin, Elaine, Brian Longhurst, Scott Mccracken, Miles Ogborn and Greg Smith. *Introducing Cultural Studies.* London: Pearson, 2010. Print.

Bande, Usha and Anshu Kaushal. Ed. *Violence in Media and Society: Literature, Film and TV.* Jaipur: Rawat Publication, 2011. Print.

Bandyopadhyay, Samik. Introduction. *Collected Plays of Mahesh Elkunchwar Vol. I.* By Elkunchwar. New Delhi: 2009. Print.

Bedre, R. T & Kadam. S. N., ed. *Reflection of the Changing Indian Society in Indian English Drama.* Narwadi: New Man Publication, 2013. Print.

Bhawe, Pushpa. *Rang Natakache.* Pune: Rajhans Prakashan, 2012. Print.

Blackshaw, Tony. *Zygmunt Bauman.* Abingdon: Routledge. 2005. Print.

Bradford, Richard. *Crime Fiction: A Very Short Introduction.* Oxford: Oxford University Press, 2015. Print.

Brownmiller, Susan. *Against Our Will: Men, Women and Rape.* New York: Fawcett Columbine, 1975. Print.

Burton, Neel. *The Meaning of Madness.* Pune: Mehta Publishing House, 2010. Print.

Carlson, Marvin. *Theatre: A Very Short Introduction.* Oxford: Oxford University Press, 2014. Print.

Chakroborty, Kaustav, ed. *Indian Drama in English.* New Delhi: PHI Learning Pvt. Ltd., 2011. Print.

Clark, Ramsey, Thomas Ehrlich Reifer and Haifa Zangana. *The Torturer in the Mirro.* New York: Seven Stories Press, 2010. Print.

Cusack, Catherine. *Theatre and Violence.* London: Palgrave Mcmillan, 2013. Print.

Dattani, Mahesh. *Collected Plays. Vol. II.* New Delhi: Penguin Books India, 2005. Print.

Deshpande, G.P., ed. *Modern Indian Drama: An Anthology.* New Delhi: Sahitya Akademi, 2000. Print.

Dhande, Chandrakant. *Marathi Natyasamiksha.* Aurangabad: Kirti Prakashan, 2006. Print.

Dow, Paul. E. *Criminology in Literature.* New York: Longman, 1980. Print.

Duncker, Patricia. *Hallucinating Foucault.* London: Picador, 1996. Print.

Durrant, Will. *The Pleasures of Philosophy.* New York: Simon and Schuster, 1953. Print.

Easthope, Antony. *The Unconscious.* Oxon: Routledge, 2009. Print.

Elkunchwar, Mahesh, Ashish Rajadhyksha, S. Bondyopadhya and S. Arvikar. *Batchit Mahesh Elkunchwaranshi.* Pune: Rajhans Prakashan. 2008. Print.

Fanon, Franz. *The Wretched of the Earth.* Harmondsworth: Penguin Books, 1965. Print.

Foucault, Michel. *Discipline and Punish: The Birth of Prison.* Trans. Alen Sheridan, London: Penguin Books, 1977. Print.

Foucault, Michel. *The History of Sexuality. Vol. I.* New York: Vintage Books. 1990. Print.

Gill, Harjeet Singh and Bernard Pottier. Ed. *Ideas, Words and Things: French Writings in Semiology.* London: Sangam Books, 1992. Print.

Golding, William. *The Lord of the Flies.* New York: A Perigee Book. 1954. Print.

Priesley, J.B. *Art of the Dramatist.* Trans. Gole, V. H. Pune: Continental Prakashan, 1974. Print.

Goodman, Randolph. *Drama: A View from the Wings.* New York: Rinehart & Wilson, 1978. Print.

Grosz, Elizabeth. *Jaques Lacan: A Feminist Introduction.* London: Routledge, 1990. Print.

Guerin, Wilfred L., Earle Labor, Lee Morgan. *A Handbook of Critical Approaches to Literature.* New York: Oxford University Press, 2005. Print.

Gupta, V.P.. *Jean – Paul Sarte: The Mastermind of Awareness,* Delhi: Vijay Goel Publishers, 2009. Print.

Hall, Kristy. *The Stuff of Fantasy.* London: Karnac Books Ltd. 2007. Print.

Hawkes, David. *Ideology.* London: Routledge, 2007. Print.

Hinton, John. *Dying.* Harmondsworth: 1967. Print.

Hobsbawm, Eric. *The Age of Revolution 1789 – 1848.* New York: Vintage Books. 1996. Print.

Jha, Raj Kamal. *The Blue Bedspread.* London: Picador. 1999. Print

Jung, C. G. *Memories, Dreams, Reflections,* Trans. Richard and Clara Winston, New York: Vintage Books, 1989. Print.

Kamlesh. Ed. *Wada Chirebandi, Magna Talyakathi Yugant: Ek Avalokan.* Pune: Sandarbh Prakashan, 1996. Print.

Kaned, Manik. *Jagtik Rangabhumi: Pachimrang 02.* Pune: Rohan Prakashan, 2007. Print.

…, *Jagtik Rangabhumi: Purvarang 01.* Pune: Rohan Prakashan, 2007. Print.

Kulkarni, D. B. Natak: *Swaroop va Samiksha.* Pune: Padmagandha Prakashan, 2010. Print.

Kunte, Madhavi edt. *Hinsa Te Dahashatwad*. Pune: Diamond Publications, 2009. Print.

Lal, Madan. Introduction. *Collected Plays of Mahesh Elkunchwar Vol. II*. By Elkunchwar. New Delhi: (2011): xxii. Print.

Leader, Darian and Judy Groves. *Introducing Lacan*. Duxford: Icon Books, 2000. Print.

Lowen, Alexander. *Depression and the Body: The Biological Basis of Faith and Reality*. Harmondsworth: Penguin Books, 1982. Print.

Machiavelli. *The Prince*. Trans. C. E. Detmold. Kent:1997. Print.

Manohar, Madhav. *Marathi Natka Thite Ka*. Mumbai: Vasant Book Stall, 1987. Print.

Marcus, Sharon. *Fighting Bodies, Fighting Words: A Theory and Politics of Rape Prevention*. Columbia: Routledge. 2002. Print.

McKie, Linda. *Families, Violence and Social Change*. New York: Tata McGraw-Hill, 2010. Print.

Mehta, Vijaya. Foreword. *Collected Plays of Mahesh Elkunchwar Vol. I*. By Elkunchwar. New Delhi: 2011. Print.

Merchant. Hoshang. *Yarana: Gay Writings from India*. New Delhi: Penguin, 1999. Print.

Millette, Kate. *Sexual Politics*. Urbana and Chicago: University of Illinois Press, 1970. Print.

Naik, Rajive and Pravin Bhole. *Bhartiya Prayogkalancha Parichay va Itihaas: Natya*. Mumbai: Lokwangmay Gruh. 2010. Print.

Narrain, Arvind. *Queer'despised Sexuality: Law and Social Change*. Bangalore: Books for Change Pub. 2004. Print.

Narrain, Avind, and Gautham Bhan. ed. *Because I Have a Voice: Queer Politics in India*. New Delhi: Yodha Press. 2005. Print.

Nemade, Bhalchandra. *Tikaswayanwar,* Aurangabad: Saket Prakashan, 1990. Print.

Nietzsche, Friedrich Wilhelm. *Twilight of the Idols with Antichrist and Ecce Homo.* London: Wordsworth Edition Ltd., 2007. Print.

Pendhari, Supriya. *Marathi Natyasrushtitil Vidroh ani Navata.* Nagpur: Vijay Prakashan,2002. Print.

Rakesh, Mohan. *Halfway House.* New Delhi: OUP. 1990. Print.

Ramanujan, A. K. "The Indian Oedipus." *Vishnu on Freud's Desk: A Reader in Psychoanalysis and Hinduism,* ed. T.G. Vaidyanathan and Jeffery J. Kripal, New Delhi:Oxford University Press. 1999. Print.

Ratner, Carl. *Cultural Psychology: Theory and Method.* New York: Kluwer Academic/Plenum Publishers, 2002.

Rothbard, Murray N. *Eagalitarianism as a Revolt Against Nature and Other Essays.* Auburn: 2000. Print.

Rudnytsky, Peter L. *Freud and Oedipus.* New York: Columbia University Press, 1987. Print.

Salunkhe. A.H. *Astikshiromani: Charvak.* Satara: Lokayat Prakashan, 1992. Print.

Sarang, Vilas. *Wangmayin Sanskruti va Samajik Wastav,* Mumbai: Mauj Prakashan, 2011. Print.

Sartre, Jean-Paul. Preface. *The Wretched of the Earth.* by Franz Fanon. Harmondsworth: Penguin Books: (1965): 23-26. Print

Schmid, A. P. and Jongman A. J. *Political Terrorism: A New Guide to Actors, Authors, Concepts, Data Bases, Theories, and Literature.* New Brunswick: Transaction Books.2005. Print.

Scruton, Roger. *Sexual Desire.* New York: Continuum, 2006. Print.

Selden, Raman, Peter Widdowson and Peter Brooker. *A Reader's Guide to Contemporary Literary Theory.* Noida: Pearson, 2006. Print.

Shah, A. B. Ed. *The Roots of Obscenity.* Bombay: Lalvani Publishing House, 1968. Print.

Shinde, Tarabai. *Stri-Purush Tulana*. Ed. Nagnath Kottapalle. Aurangabad: Kailash Publication. 2010. Print.

Siddiqui, M.A. Sami. Ed. *Violence in Indian English Drama*. Jaipur: Vital Publication, 2013. Print.

Strauss, Levi. *The Raw and the Cooked*. Trans. John and Doreen Weightman. Plon. 1964. Print.

Sukthankar, Ashwini. *Facing the Mirror: Lesbian Writings from India*. New Delhi: Penguin, 1999. Print.

Tendulkar, Vijay. *Mi Jinkalo Mi Harlo,* Mumbai, Popular Prakashan, 1963. Print.

Thompson, Ken. *Emile Durkheim*. London: Routledge, 1982. Print.

Vhatkar, Namdeo. *Marathi Loknatya Tamasha: Kala ani Sahitya,* Kolhapur: Ajab Publications, 2010. Print.

Vatsyayana. *Kamasutra*. Trans. Richard Francis Burton. New Delhi: Penguin Evergreens, 1862. Print.

Williams, Raymond. *Marxism and Literature*. Oxford: Oxford University Press, 1977. Print.

Zizek Slovej. *Looking Awry.* Cambridge: MIT Press, 1992. Print.

…, *The Plague of Fantasies.* London: Verso, 1997. Print.

…, *Violence*. New York: Picador, 2008. Print.

Chapters in Books:

Bhagat, Datta. "Marathi Natak: 1975 to 2000." *Marathi Natak Ani Rangbhumi.* ed. Shinde, Wishwanath and Smart, Himanshu. Pune: Pratima Prakashan, 2008. Print.

Hawaldar, Pratima, "Kai Aahe Hinsachar?" *Hinsa Te Dahashatwad.* ed. Kunte, Pune: Diamond Publications, 2009. Print.

Ramanujan, A. K. "The Indian Oedipus." *Vishnu on Freud's Desk: A Reader in Psychoanalysis and Hinduism.* ed.T.G. Vaidyanathan and Jeffery J. Kripal, New Delhi:Oxford University Press. 1999. Print.

Documentary:

Zizek, Slovej. *Pervert's Guide to Cinema. www.youtube.com*, youtube, mp4, *2005*. Web. 20 May, 2010.

Journal Articles:

Barure, Somnath. "Mahesh Elkunchwar's *Old Stone Mansion* – End of Ethos." *International Journal of English Language & Translation Studies* 2:4 (2014):74. Web. 24 Oct, 2015.

Bhagwat, Hemangi. "Dalit Theatre: A Theatre of Protest". *European Academic Research* 2:1 (2014): 384. Web. 11 Oct. 2015.

Chattopadhyay, Malyaban. "A Historical Study of Ancient Indian Theatre – Communication in the Light of *Natyasastra*". *Global Media Journal* 4:2 (2013): 12. Web. 3 Oct, 2015.

Dey, Sayan. "Contribution of Mahesh Elkunchwar in the Evolution of Post-Colonial Marathi Theatre: Tracing the Theatrical History". *International Journal of Humanities and Social Science Invention* 3:3 (2014): 18. Web.16 Aug, 2015.

Dey, Sayan. "(Dis)locating Theoritical Catachresis in Mahesh Elkunchwar: A Playwright's Re-creative Journey from the Western Pages to the Practical World." *International Journal of English Language, Literature and Humanities* 2:10 (2015):287. Web. 16, Oct, 2015.

Elkunchwar, Mahesh. *Yatanaghar*. Mumbai: Mauj Prakashan, 1997. Print. Elkunchwar, Mahesh and Anjum Katyal. "A Playwright of Human Relationships: An Interview with Mahesh Elkunchwar." *Seagull Theatre Quarterly* 22. 1999. Print.

Jahagirdar, Chandrashekhar. "Marathi Drama After 1960." *Haritham* 5 (1995):66. Print.

Khan, Nazneen. "Myriad Themes Immaculately Crafted in a Family Saga: Mahesh Elkunchwar's *Wada Trilogy.*" *The Quest,* 28:1 2014): 40. Print.

Kulkarni, Purnima. "Subalterns Speak in Mahesh Elkunchwar's *Holi*". *Contemporary Discourse* 6:1 (2015): 219. Web. 20 Oct, 2015.

Mathi, Nirai.S. "Mahashweta Devi, the Rebel Playwright of Mother of 1084." *The Literary Criterion* 3&4 (2007): 33. Print

Mohan, Indra T.M.J.. "Post – Colonial Writing – Trends in English Drama". *The Indian Review of World Literature in English* 2:2 (2006): 5. Web.2 Jan, 2015.

Mohanty, Prafull. K. "Freedom as Identity: The Literature of Rising". *Indian Literature, Sahitya Akademi's Bi-Monthly Journal* 1. (2009): 220. Print.

Nadkarni, Dnyaneshwar. "Elkunchwar's 'Party'." *Enact,* (1976):27. Print. Palla, Venkat Murali. "Thematic Study of Mahesh Elkunchwar's *Flower of Blood*". *International Journal of Multidisciplinary Educational Research* 3:7 (2014) 227. Web. 19 Oct, 2015.

Primlyn, A. Linda. "The Sound of Silence in Mahesh Elkunchwar's Plays: *The Pond* and *Party.*" *The Atalantic Literary Review Quarterly* 14:3 (2013): 89. Print.

Ram, Mohan, "Five Years After Naxalbari." *Economic and Political Weekly 7* Web (1972): 1471.

Rose, Beulah. "A Solution to the Question of Absurdity in Elkunchwar's *'Reflection'.*" *The Quest* 8:2 (1994): 27. Print.

Shirly, Sidney. "Sexuality Versus Psychology: A Study of Mahesh Elkunchwar's *Garbo* and *Desire in the Rocks*". *Journal of English Language and Literature 2:1*(2015): 124. Web. 12 Oct, 2015. Print.

Shulman, Alix Kats. "Sex and Power: Sexual Bases of Radical Feminism." *Signs* 5:4 (1980): 591. JSTOR. Web. June, 2011.

Thokor, Daxa. "Social Issues in *Where There's a Will*". *Galaxy: International Multidisciplinary Research Journal* 1:1 (2012): 2. Web. 10 Jan, 2015.

Zizek, Slovej. "Language, Violence and Nonviolence." *International Journal of Zizek Studies* 2:3 (2008): 01. Web. 21 Jan, 2014.

Magazine Articles:

Mittal, Tusha. "How a Deaf Ear is Turning Plughshares to Swords". *Tehelka* 44 (2009): 30. Print.

Reviews:

Ambedkar, B. R. "Mr. Russell and the Reconstruction of Society." Rev. of *Principles of Social Reconstruction, Journal of the Indian Economic Society* 01 July, 1918: 16. Print.

Deshpande, Sudhnva. "The Radical Conservative." Rev. of *Collected Plays of Mahesh Elkunchwar, The Book Review* 20.4. Sept, 2010: 31. Print.

Jain, Kirti. "Chronicles of a Disturbing Time." Rev. of *The Collected Plays of Satish Alekar: Collected Plays of Mahesh Elkunchwar, The Little Magazine*, 8.1 June, 2009: 186. Print.

Rathi, Giridhar. "The Indian Crucible." Rev. of *Pratibimb Aur Aatmakathaa. The Book Review,* 20.4 Nov, 1996: 35. Print.

Singh, Neelam Man. "Spearheading Modernism." Rev. of *Collected Plays of Mahesh Elkunchwar Vol.II, The Book Review* 36.12. Dec, 2012: 25. Print.

Dissertations:

"On the Principles of Political Violence and Anti-Fascist Action" Diss. University of Manchester, Web. 19 July, 2015.